CW00969067

Outline of Clinical Diagnosis in Sheep

This volume is dedicated to shepherds

'No man is closer to the beast he tends,
Nor, idle, savours such contented days;
No man more blessed free' . . .

The Land   V. Sackville-West

'Shepherds and stars are quiet with the hills,
There is a bond between the men who go
From youth about the business of the earth,
The earth they serve, their cradle and their grave;
Stars with the seasons alter; only he
Who wakeful follows the pricked revolving sky,
Turns concordant with the earth while others sleep;
To him the dawn is punctual; to him
The quarters of the year no empty name.

The Land   V. Sackville-West

Outline of Clinical Diagnosis in Sheep

J. C. Hindson BVSc, MRCVS
North Park Veterinary Group, North Tawton, Devon

Agnes C. Winter BVSc, DSHP, MRCVS
Department of Veterinary Clinical Science,
University of Liverpool

'My flocks feed not,
My ewes breed not,
My rams speed not,
All is amiss.'
Sonnets to Sundry Notes of Music   Shakespeare

WRIGHT
London   Boston   Singapore   Sydney   Toronto   Wellington

Wright
is an imprint of Butterworth Scientific

 PART OF REED INTERNATIONAL P.L.C.

First published 1990

© **Butterworth & Co. (Publishers) Ltd, 1990**

British Library Cataloguing in Publication Data

Hindson, J. C.
  Outline of clinical diagnosis in sheep.
  1. Livestock. Sheep diseases
  I. Title   II. Winter, Agnes C.
  636.30896

ISBN 0-7236-1187-4

Library of Congress Cataloging in Publication Data

Hindson, J. C.
  Outline of clinical diagnosis in sheep / J.C. Hindson,
  Anges C. Winter.
     p.   cm.
  Includes bibliographical references.
  ISBN 0-7236-1187-4
  1. Sheep–Diseases–Diagnosis.   I. Winter, Agnes C.   II. Title.
  [DNLM: 1. Sheep Diseases–diagnosis–outlines. SF 968 H662o]
  SF968.H56   1990   89-70642
  636.3'089'6075–dc20   CIP

Laserset by Scribe Design, Gillingham, Kent
Printed and bound in Great Britain by Courier International Ltd, Tiptree, Essex

Acknowledgements

We acknowledge with thanks the help given to us by many people during the gestation of this book. In particular, we would like to thank Professor Michael Clarkson, Department of Veterinary Clinical Science, University of Liverpool; David Byrne, North Park Veterinary Group, North Tawton; Judith Charnley, Colne, and Neil Spedding, Ripon for helpful comments on the completed manuscript. Advice on individual chapters has been given by other colleagues in the Faculty of Veterinary Science, University of Liverpool, particularly Geoff Skeritt and Penny Lazarus, and also by members of the Veterinary Investigation Service. Thanks are also due to Gary Hynes, Department of Veterinary Clinical Science, University of Liverpool, who took the photographs. Finally, we wish to thank our spouses, Mary and Tom, who kept bodies, souls and houses together during the writing process!

Contents

1 Introduction

Successful animal health care, be it for disease, welfare or economic considerations, rests on the triple pillars of diagnosis, prognosis and treatment. Without a high degree of accuracy in the first, prognosis becomes a lottery, and treatment may well degenerate into a dependence on 'shot-gun' or 'spray' therapy. This text has been prepared in an attempt to assist the clinician to answer accurately the question – 'why are my sheep too fat?, too thin? too dead?' – this being the starting point in most investigations. The hope is that, by separating diagnosis from treatment and basing the sections on signs rather than systems, the clinician may more readily arrive at a successful solution to the problems presented by sheep keepers.

No attempt has been made to include every possible condition which could occur at very low incidence – 'the once in a lifetime type', since this would make the text simply confusing, and make the selection of probable causes difficult.

It is impossible to produce a definitive text for any changing science. In particular, laboratory diagnostic techniques are progressing rapidly – note the introduction of DNA probes. This text is therefore based on widely accepted and commercially available techniques, commonly used at the time of going to press.

Special difficulties of clinical diagnosis in the sheep

'For the sheep when well is often times capricious and when sick does wish to die.' Anon

Diagnosis of the cause of a deviation from normal in any species of livestock makes special demands on the combined knowledge and experience of the clinician. The sheep does, however, present its own special problems. The simple process of isolating the patient from its group frequently induces sufficient stress to mask any behavioural change, which is often the first indicator to the shepherd of an abnormality. Confirmation of the owner's original complaint may not, therefore, be open to the clinician; indeed behavioural change as a primary indicator of disease cannot be relied on. The sheep, in common with some other domesticated species and with the majority of 'wild' species, exhibits a passive or 'dumb' response when unpleasant external stimuli reach a certain threshold. Beyond this point, no further response will be produced even to painful stimulation and diagnosis must be based on other means. This attitude may also occur during the terminal phases of disease and is the probable origin of the conviction that all sheep have a death wish!

In the diagnosis of disease in most animals, variations from normal in respiratory rate, pulse rate and temperature are commonly used early in the diagnostic procedure. None of these are of great value in the sheep, except in the very young lamb where abnormal temperature is significant. Pulse rate may be of little diagnostic value, as catching and handling usually cause a marked increase, except in animals well accustomed to regular handling. Since respiration is the primary route of heat loss, wide variations in the respiratory rate occur depending on ambient temperature, length of fleece, pregnancy and other factors. Similarly, the body temperature may be elevated above that generally recognized as the 'normal', particularly in hot weather in animals carrying substantial amounts of fleece.

The clinician must be aware of these factors, and subject any observations of deviations from 'normal' to serious question, not placing reliance on body temperature, heart or respiratory rate alone in the absence of other signs. The value of auscultation is also limited by the presence of fleece cover, which masks the details of abnormal respiratory and heart sounds.

Routine for clinical examination

It is important even for the experienced clinician to have a routine procedure for the investigation of any problems. There is a very real temptation to take short cuts either based on first impressions or based on previous experience of what may well mistakenly be assumed to be an identical incident.

When carrying out the initial history taking perhaps the most essential requirement is that we keep an open mind, and of great importance is a realization that the complaint the client presents may not in fact be the real one. An animal presented by the sheep keeper as suffering from constipation, for example, is most unlikely to be so, and in all probability the problem lies in a different body system. In addition, knowledge of the farm history and the client may be just as much a hindrance as a help if this narrows the range of possibilities at too early a stage.

In the case of investigation of disease in the sheep, the postmortem examination (PME) is likely to play an important role. Thus a routine for this technique in both the adult and the neonate, together with details of sample taking, form important parts of the text.

The following list is a suggested sequence for the examination of an individual or group, and for the building up of the necessary information on which to base both a diagnosis and prognosis (see also Figure 1.1).

(1) The owner's complaint.
(2) Description of the patient(s) – age and sex.
(3) Number affected – many animals, a few, or single individual.

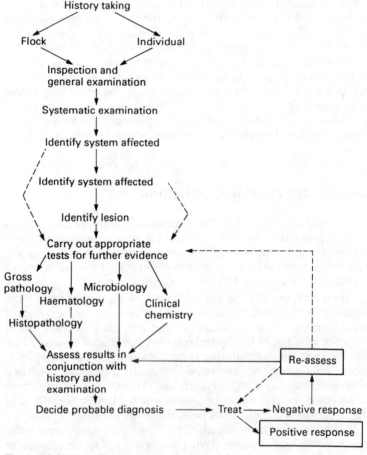

Figure 1.1 Steps in diagnostic procedure

(4) History of this incident, and in the past.
(5) Knowledge of the farm, client and area.
(6) Inspection.
(7) Systematic examination.
(8) PME where applicable.
(9) Specimen taking.
(10) Laboratory examination and results.
(11) Diagnosis.
(12) Prognosis.

Examination check list

The following is a suggested routine for a full clinical examination of a sheep. Obviously not all cases will require such a comprehensive examination, therefore any sections irrelevant to a particular case should be omitted.

Owner   Date
Animal/s identity
Sex
Age

Inspection
    appearance
    behaviour
    gait
    appetite
    faeces
    fleece
    respiration   ⎫ bearing in mind
Examination   ⎬ limitations
    temperature, normal range 39–40°C   ⎭ as mentioned
    pulse
    condition score 1–5
    fleece/skin
    head
        position
        nostrils – discharge, breath
        eyes – conjunctiva, cornea, pupil, discharge
        mouth – lips, teeth, jaws, breath
    chest
        auscultate, palpate over heart
        wheelbarrow test
    abdomen
        size, shape, auscultate, palpate, ballot

urinary system – urine, urethra (male)
external genitalia
    male – scrotum, testicles, prepuce, penis
    female – vulva, mammary glands
limbs – feet, joints
nervous system
full neurological examination if necessary.

Interpretation of clinical signs

In this book, each chapter tackles a problem or sign as it is likely to be presented by the client. In the forefront of the veterinarians's mind when carrying out the initial discussions will be the fact that there exists a range of clinical entities which have an obvious age distribution . . . lamb dysentery limited to the neonate, coccidiosis to the young lamb, and pregnancy toxaemia to the pregnant adult ewe, for example. For this reason the text has been subdivided in certain sectors into age categories, to reduce the amount of text the reader must follow. Similarly, certain conditions are definitely group or flock problems.

2 Suboptimal reproductive performance (SORP)

Low mating activity
High rate of returns to service
Individual female infertility
Delayed returns to service
Artificial manipulation of breeding season
  problems
Artificial manipulation of prolificacy
  problems
Suboptimal lamb numbers
Inadequate lamb birth weights
Barren ewes

In most flocks, at least 60% of the profitability is a function of number of lambs reared together with stocking rate. Since feeding the ewe accounts for some 90% of total feed costs in the case of the production of single lambs, and in excess of 80% in the case of twins, it is entirely understandable and right that the client be concerned by poor flock reproductive performance, and that solutions are urgently demanded from the veterinarian. Suboptimal reproductive performance will, therefore, be one of the most common complaints with which the veterinarian will be presented. In turn, the clinician must accept the responsibility to investigate, but will need great tact in presenting the solutions.

The client will probably assume in the first instance that the cause must be some 'dread' disease, since that absolves him or her from any blame or reflection on the management of the flock. Unfortunately for the clinician, this problem will be presented most often at lambing time when the cause may have existed some 5 months previously. Identifying what went wrong will probably be extremely difficult, and no immediate solution can be offered. The final complication is that, with very few exceptions, the cause will not be some 'dread' disease, but will frequently be multifactorial and difficult to identify with total conviction.

Suboptimal reproductive performance can be caused by the following:

- Low ovulation rates
- Low conception rates
- Early fetal loss/reabsorption
- Late fetal death
- Abortion
- Stillbirth
- Dystocia and prolapse
- Poor mothering ability
- Male infertility

Table 2.1 highlights common causes of the problem. Abortion, dystocia and prolapse, and male infertility are dealt with in separate chapters (see chapters 3, 4 and 5).

It is essential that we start with definitions of reproductive performance. This must be considered not only in terms of total output, but also must take into account the duration of the lambing period, the litter size, numbers of ewes in any group failing to breed, and the numbers of ewes in any group failing to rear lambs which they have carried to term.

Table 2.1 Suboptimal reproductive performance

Problem	Common causes	
Anoestrus	Season Nutrition Lactation Pregnancy	
Low ovulation rate	Season Nutrition Breed	
Failure to conceive	Male infertility	
Low conception rate	Male:female ratio Nutrition Social effects	
Embryonic loss	Genetic ⎤ Chromosomal ⎦ Nutrition – very high, very low Stress	
Early fetal death	Infection – toxoplasma, border disease Nutrition – sudden change Stress	
Late fetal loss	Infection (all infectious causes of abortion) Placental insufficiency (fetal overload)	
Intrapartum fetal death	Management Dystocia	
Postpartum death	Dystocia ⎤ Management ⎥ Maternal factors ⎬ Environmental factors ⎥ Infection ⎦	Dystocia – mismothering – exposure – starvation complex

Although male infertility is considered separately, the possibility of ram involvement in any problem must always be kept in mind.

Irrespective of breed, season or location there can only be one true indicator of reproductive output, the lambing percentage, i.e. *the number of lambs reared per 100 ewes put to the ram.* This may be a wide and rather ruthless definition and does include losses other than those strictly under consideration under the heading of SORP, but any other definition is only deluding the breeder.

When deciding what constitutes an acceptable flock performance, it is sensible to take into consideration contemporary losses in similar flocks particularly in adverse seasons or environment, otherwise much time may be wasted looking for other causes which do not exist.

There are wide variations in acceptable output, not only between breeds, but within any one breed due to genetic factors. There will also be wide variations due to environmental factors. For example, output from the Scottish Blackface in high hill conditions may be as low as 60%, but the same ewes under lowland conditions might produce up to 150%.

The first essential exercise is to establish the true output upon which the client is basing the complaint, and to compare that with some known standard for the breed, season and environment.

These standards must be realistic, and not taken from breed propaganda or other biased sources. The Meat and Livestock Commission (MLC) Flockplan records form a firm basis on which to begin comparisons, giving average and top third performances for a wide variety of breeds and crosses in a range of environmental conditions.

Some examples of national figures and targets:

Ewe deaths – national range is 4–10%, target is 2%.

Barren ewes – national range is 4–10%, target is 2%.

(The higher figures apply to hill flocks which are unlikely to be able to achieve a very low target in adverse environmental conditions.)

Number of ewes mated during first cycle – target is 80%.

This figure is required to achieve a maximum duration of lambing for optimum output and management efficiency of 4 weeks. This may seem to be a peripheral factor, but is regarded rightly by MLC as indicative of good matching of breed, season, environment and nutrition for maximum ovulation and conception rates.

The starting point in any flock investigation will be the stage in the breeding cycle at which the complaint originates, and whether the problem involves individual or many ewes, a whole group, or all groups.

Problems during the mating period

Early in mating period, low mating activity

- Check for possible pregnancy (Doppler pregnancy detector can be used from 30 days, scanner from 50 days).
- Check ewe and season compatibility, e.g.
  Dorset Horns will breed anytime
  Suffolks are early breeders

Mules mid-season
Texels mid-late season
Welsh Mountain late season
Soay limited to three cycles starting in November.

● Check nutrition of ewes (Figure 2.1). Condition score (minimum of 10–15% if large group) – see Table 2.2 for effect of condition score on litter size.
Metabolic profile if necessary.
● Check weaning to mating interval (minimum 5 weeks).
● Check rams – breed, number, soundness.
● Check for ewe immaturity (ewe lambs will not begin cycling until several weeks after mature ewes of same breed).

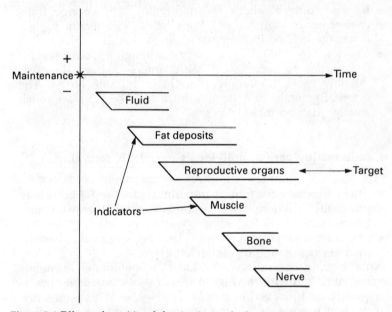

Figure 2.1 Effects of nutritional deprivation on body tissues

Full mating activity, high return rate

● Check rams' fertility (see Chapter 5).
● Check male/female ratio; 1:40 recommended for mature male, 1:25 for ram lamb, 1:10 if synchronized.

- Check for correct harness application (these have been known to be put on incorrectly so interfering physically with mating, or too tightly causing pain)
- Check for presence of brisket lesions – may cause pain.

High return rate with vaginal discharge

- Check for infectious vaginitis or balanoposthitis.
- If sponges were used, check hygiene precautions.

Late in mating period, individuals not mated

- Check for pregnancy (lost or worn crayon).
- If synchronized, check for non-removal of sponge (may require use of vaginoscope). Presence of characteristic vaginal discharge is good indicator of retained sponge.
- Check for congenital abnormality – although it is not usual for freemartins to occur as in cattle, intersex sheep do exist, possibly more commonly from high multiple births. The external genitalia may be abnormal, and the teats are much smaller than normal females.

Late in mating period, individuals repeatedly returning to service

- Check for excessive fatness in perineal area, or fat tail – may physically interfere with mating. Tail wool may require trimming.
- Check for trauma from previous lambing – vaginal adhesions (digital examination or vaginoscope).

Note: Examination of the individual ewe is of limited economic value, although with the high prices of exotic breeds it may be requested and justified in some animals. Use of a vaginoscope may allow examination of the vagina and cervix for anatomical defects or evidence of trauma. With high value animals, use of a laparoscope will allow examination of ovaries and fallopian tubes.

Late in mating period, many not mated

- Check validity of complaint – harness fitting, crayon loss.
- Check for pregnancy.

- Check age; if ewe lambs, possible immaturity, if shearlings, possible social factors, e.g. breed factors, likes and dislikes of rams.
- Check true age, may be late lambs therefore late to cycle.
- Check body condition score – too fat, too thin.
- Check weaning date – lactation effect.
- Check rams – lameness, inexperience, low libido, small ram lambs expected to mate large ewes.

Late in mating period, high rate of returns to service

- Check male/female ratio.
- Recheck male – sudden infertility, exhaustion, trauma, infections.
- Check for stress, e.g. dipping.

High rate of returns more than 30 days after first mating

- Check for stress, e.g. dipping.
- Check for sudden nutritional stress.
- Check for toxoplasmosis – rising titres.
- Check for border disease – rising titres.

Special problems associated with manipulation of the breeding season or prolificacy

Many sheep keepers have had disappointing results from first attempts to either synchronize or advance the breeding season. The advent of hormone or immunologically induced methods of increasing lambing percentage has also produced far from optimum results in some units. Since the financial input for such techniques is significant, requests for explanations and avoidance of repetition are frequently met. As these are prescription-only medicine (POM) products obtainable only from the veterinary surgeon, careful advice on their use should have been given at the time of supply. Thus any discussion about unsatisfactory results should rightly be directed at the clinician initially.

When any such product is supplied, the client must be advised that the instruction sheet for the drug must at all times be followed carefully. Any other course will preclude any complaint to the manufacturer from having any validity.

The following products are commonly in use:
for forward extension of the breeding season:
    intravaginal sponges + PMSG
    (melatonin – availability commercially is imminent)
for synchronization within the normal breeding season:
    intravaginal sponges
    prostaglandins may be used but may have poor results
for increasing prolificacy:
    immunization (Fecundin)
    intravaginal sponges + PMSG

Forward advancement of breeding season, ewes not mating after sponge removal

- Check breed of ewe and realistic advancement achievable. Treatment is only really worthwhile in transition from anoestrum when some ovarian activity is beginning.
- Check ram breed, libido and fertility. Seasonal breeding patterns occur in some breeds more than others. Dorset, Friesland and Finn are very early, down breeds early, Texel and hill breeds late.

Poor conception rate to synchronized first service in advanced or normal breeding season

- Check timing of ram introduction – too early? too late? Recommended time is 48 h after sponge removal. If introduced too early, rams may be exhausted before period of maximum fertility, if too late, will miss fertile period.
- Check ewe to ram ratio, 10:1 recommended.
- Check fertility of rams.
- Check technique and hygiene of sponge application.
- Check condition of ewes, plus weaning to sponging interval.

Within normal breeding season, low mating activity after sponge removal

- Check rams, numbers, libido and fertility.
- Check timing of ram introduction.
- Check for lost sponges (alters timing of oestrus).
- Check for retained sponges (prevents oestrus).

Too high a litter size

● Check PMSG dosage

Note: Variations in the dose response for PMSG are notorious and are the rule rather than the exception. Very high doses may have a negative effect. The normal dose is 500–750 units.

Poor response to Fecundin

● Check breed suitability.
● Check body condition and nutrition at mating and throughout pregnancy.
● Check timing of injections (primary course is given 8 and 4 weeks before mating, in subsequent years single dose 4 weeks before mating).

Note: The best response may be expected from ewes with a lambing percentage normally in the range 120–170%. An increase of 20–25% may be expected and is required to justify the costs, which are significant. Breeds with a normally low lambing percentage may respond with increased numbers of lambs, but with low birth weights, possibly due to limited placental capacity, or with adequate weights but poor lactation capacity. Breeds with high prolificacy will respond but with a risk of litters with low viability.

It is essential that these factors are in the forefront of any discussion about the possible introduction of this technique.

Suboptimal lamb numbers

The first step must be to establish whether the complaint is justified by comparing production with similar units, the same breed, season and region.

As previously stated, any problems investigated at this time will reflect events which have taken place some months before and the effects of any advice will only emerge some months in the future. It will be difficult, most of all, to establish the true nutritional status of the flock at the time of mating and conception. In addition, the clinician must at all times be aware of the client's wish to escape any 'blame' for the problem.

If it is established that the complaint is genuine, then the detailed analysis must establish whether the problem is: (a) low litter size throughout the flock, (b) normal litter size with a high barren ewe rate, (c) high perinatal lamb mortality (see chapter 8).

Low litter size

Individual animals consistently producing low numbers will not be noticed in an otherwise normal flock unless detailed recording is carried out. Individual pedigree persistent low producers may involve a genetic factor. The tendency to buy well grown ram lambs for breeding means that, in the absence of records to the contrary, these animals are often singles, which perpetuates low litter size.

Many ewes producing low litter size

- Check age of affected animals; immaturity, old age.
- Check familial relationship if known – owner selection for other characteristics may be selecting for low fecundity, e.g. use of single-born ram lambs as above.
- Check for body score at tupping – poor condition at mating gives low ovulation rates, poor conception rates (see Table 2.2).
- Check for nutrition through pregnancy – low conception rate plus high fetal loss or reabsorption – check placentae for evidence.
- Check for evidence of toxoplasmosis or border disease (see chapter 3).
- Check for stress at critical stages of gestation. May be possible to demonstrate growth retardation lines in long bones as evidence of check.

Normal litter size, many barren ewes

- Check age of barren ewes – immaturity or old age.
- Check breed of barren ewes – late maturing breed, social factors – different breed from ram, breed incompatibility.
- Check duration of mating period – too early ram withdrawal for some ewes because of breed or season incompatibility.
- Check weaning dates of barren group – lactation effect.
- Check for evidence of unobserved abortions – border disease and toxoplasmosis.

Table 2.2 Effect of body condition score on lambing percentage

Type of ewe	Lambs born per 100 ewes put to ram Condition score						
	1	1.5	2	2.5	3	3.5	4
Hill ewes							
Scottish Blackface		79			162		
Gritstone (hill)			75	103	119	109	
Welsh Mountain	60	65	105	116	123		
Swaledale		78	133	140	156		
Lowland ewes							
Gritstone (lowland)				132	154	173	
Masham				167	181	215	
Mule			149	166	178	194	192
Greyface			147	163	176	189	184
Welsh Halfbred		126	139	150	164	172	
Scottish Halfbred			148	170	183	217	202

(From MLC *Feeding the Ewe*, 1981)

- Check for evidence of concurrent disease or stress during pregnancy causing fetal loss.
- Check if are recent introductions – rejects from other units

Normal litter size, inadequate birth weights

- Check for nutrition in early pregnancy (inadequate placentation).
- Check body condition score – inadequate feeding in late pregnancy has always been assumed to be a major influence. This is now open to question.
- Check for infectious agent (see chapter 3).

See also chapter 8, perinatal lamb losses.

Investigations required before next season irrespective of the cause of this episode

- Check owner knowledge of effects of nutrition throughout the breeding cycle.
- Check ram management, owner knowledge of good ram preparation.

● Check body condition score at weaning and select fat or thin groups for appropriate feeding in dry period (see Tables 2.1 and 2.2).

Note: On maximum sustainable nutritional inputs, it takes 3 weeks to gain 1/2 condition score.

● Check nutrition at critical times (condition score, pasture and feed assessment, metabolic profile if necessary), especially 6–8 weeks pretupping when on standard intake.

● Check for evidence of specific infections – abortion profile of representative group if indicated.

● Check for parasite control.

● Check for possible micronutrient deficiency. Copper deficiency is not thought to have any effect on conception rates but can cause lambs of low viability; selenium deficiency may have an effect on reproduction although this is not proven.

Provide (a) record keeping facilities, (b) nutrition guidance, (c) disease control plan, (d) facility for prompt investigation and diagnosis as problems arise.

3 Abortion

Infectious causes
  Enzootic
  Toxoplasmosis
  Border disease
  Campylobacteriosis
  Salmonellosis
  Listeriosis
  Other minor/sporadic causes
Non-infectious causes
  Nutrition
  Stress
  Concurrent disease
Guide to diagnosis

Abortion itself clearly does not present any problem of diagnosis. It is in the investigation of the cause or causes of an individual, or more usually, a flock problem that the clinician will be involved. Abortion should be regarded as part of the total picture of suboptimal reproductive performance, even though the sheep keeper will present it as a separate problem. It is important to remember that many of the infectious causes of abortion in sheep constitute a zoonosis risk, and that care in handling abortion material is necessary. In particular, enzootic (chlamydial) abortion and *Toxoplasma* abortion are serious risks to pregnant women, and advice to this effect should always be given to the client.

Definitions used in this text

Abortion – the expulsion before full term of a fetus which is incapable of independent life.

Premature birth – the expulsion before full term of a fetus which is capable of independent life.

Stillbirth – the expulsion of a dead full term fetus.

Gestation length – although the usually accepted length is 147 days, it is important to recognize that there are individual and breed variations, with a range of 140–150 days to be expected.

Although expulsion of a dead fetus before term is the usual evidence of abortion, during any abortion episode some fetuses may be carried to term, yet be infected, and some may be carried to term and be fully viable. It is also important to recognize that abortion incidents may be multifactorial, not only in terms of infectious agents, but also involving nutritional and management factors. These may be additive; for example, inadequate maternal nutrition may be the critical factor which changes a mild infective placentitis into terminal interference with the life support mechanisms of the fetus.

The clinician must at all times be aware that the establishment of a causal factor early in the investigation of an abortion outbreak does not end the requirement for any further concern with that episode. In addition, it should be recognized that the advice required where mixed infections such as enzootic abortion of ewes (EAE) and toxoplasmosis are diagnosed may be contradictory.

What comprises an abortion problem?

Premature births occasionally occur in all flocks, but where more than 2% of lambs are born outside the normal gestational variation, it must be presumed that some factor is present which is jeopardizing fetal survival. The owner's complaint must be treated as a matter of urgency and a full investigation initiated if an early diagnosis is to be achieved and losses reduced to a minimum. Whilst abortion storms in sheep never reach the catastrophic proportions of the initial brucellosis storms in cattle, losses of up to 50% have been recorded after the first exposure of a totally 'naive' flock to a new infectious agent: 20–30% will be a more usual proportion even during the initial storm, whilst 5–10% may well occur during chronic flock infection in seasons following that in which the infection was first introduced. The degree of loss will not act as a guide to the type of infection, but only to the presence of a chronic or new infection. Sudden change to this incidence will often indicate the addition of a further cause to an existing pattern. The stage during gestation at which abortion takes place will also not be a guide to the specific cause, but only in some cases a possible guide to the timing of infection or nutritional stress. Finally, gross pathology will often be unhelpful except in the case of EAE and toxoplasmosis.

Causes of ovine abortion

Infectious

Chlamydia – *Chlamydia psittaci* – Enzootic abortion (EAE)
Protozoon – *Toxoplasma gondii* – Toxoplasmosis
Virus – *Pestivirus* – Border disease
Bacteria
    Campylobacter foetus ⎱ Campylobacteriosis
    foetus   ⎰ (Vibriosis)
    Salmonella spp. – Salmonellosis
        S. abortus ovis
        S. dublin
        S. typhimurium
        S. montevideo
        S. arizonae
    Miscellaneous *Salmonella* spp.
    Listeria monocytogenes — Listeriosis
    Bacillus licheniformis
    (*Brucella abortus*)
Rickettsia – *Cytocetes phagocytophilia* — Tickborne fever
           Coxiella burneti — Q fever
Fungus – *Aspergillus fumigatus* — Aspergillosis

Claviceps purpurea — Ergotism
Mycotoxins
Note: Some of these infectious agents are primarily placento-
trophic, e.g. *Chlamydia, Toxoplasma, S. abortus ovis, S. montevideo.*
Others cause more generalized disease with abortion the result
of septicaemia, e.g. *S. typhimurium, S. dublin*, tickborne fever.

Non-infectious

The following factors have been implicated, and should be
considered if infectious causes are eliminated.
Inadequate nutrition
Pregnancy toxaemia
Stress
  poor handling
  vaccination
  transport
  dog worry
Concurrent disease
  pasteurellosis
  chronic fluke
*Of these many causes of ovine abortion, by far the most important are
Chlamydia and Toxoplasma which account for over 40% and over 35%
respectively of all diagnosed incidents.* A positive diagnosis of an
infectious cause only results with material from about 50% of
incidents submitted to veterinary investigation centres, but it
does not follow that the remaining 50% are not due to
infections. Inadequate or unsuitable material may have been
submitted, or tests to identify more unusual causal agents not
carried out, or fragile organisms may not survive the journey to
the laboratory.

Investigation of an outbreak (Figure 3.1)

*It is essential that the owner retain all possible material and that it be as
fresh as possible, so that the clinician is in a position to choose such
samples as will maximize the chance of an early accurate diagnosis.
Samples should be submitted from a minimum of 10% of affected ewes,
preferably more, and if abortions continue over a prolonged lambing
time, a check should be made at intervals to make sure that different
agents are not operating.*

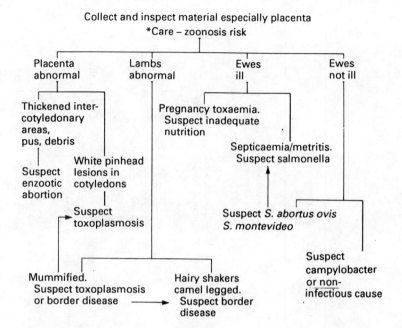

Figure 3.1 Multiple abortions

Material required varies for different agents but the following material should be obtained in every investigation:

- Dead fetuses (or fetal stomach contents and pleural fluid in vacutainers plus piece of fetal liver).
- Placenta (including cotyledons).
- Vaginal swab (if placenta not available).

Aborting ewes should be marked for later identification and sampling if necessary, and should be isolated from both pregnant and non-pregnant sheep until the cause is established.

Table 3.1 Abortion – diagnostic aids

Type	Gross pathology Placenta	Fetus	Concurrent maternal disease	Laboratory material required	Tests
Epidemic/major causes					
Chlamydia	+++	–	–	Placenta, [fetal skin swab] Blood/serum Maternal	Smear CFT ($\geq \frac{1}{64}$ is +ve)
Toxoplasma	+++	± Mummification	–	Placenta, fetal pleural fluid	LAT IFAT IHA ELISA Histology
Campylobacter	–	± Liver lesions	–	Placenta, fetal stomach contents Maternal Blood/serum	Smear culture CFT
Salmonella	–	–	– (*S. montevideo S. abortus ovis*) +++ Other spp.	Placenta, fetal stomach contents Blood/serum Maternal	Smear culture SAT
Border disease	–	++ Characteristic lambs or mummification	–	Fetus – blood, brain, spleen, lymph nodes	Virus isolation IFAT Histology

Sporadic/minor causes					
Listeriosis	−	+ Sawdust liver	++ Neurological disease within flock	Placenta / Fetus	Histology, culture
Leptospirosis	−	−	+ Milk drop	Maternal blood/serum	HAT (paired sera)
Mycotic	++	±	−	Placenta / Fetal stomach contents	Smear, histology
Q fever	−	−	±	Placenta / Maternal blood/serum	Smear, serology to distinguish from *Chlamydia*
Tickborne fever	−	−	±	Maternal blood/serum	Smear, HAT, known tick area

CFT = complement fixation test
HAT = haemagglutination test
IFAT = indirect fluorescent antibody test
IHA = indirect haemagglutination
LAT = latex agglutination test
SAT = serum agglutination test

Note: Since dystocia and metritis will be common sequelae of any individual case of abortion, septicaemia may occur as a secondary feature.

Table 3.2 Timing of infection in relation to time of abortion

Organism	Minimum time infection to abortion	Likely source
Chlamydia	6 weeks Usually infection one lambing season, abortion next season, but infection and abortion possible in same season if lambing prolonged	Infected ewe Placenta Fetal fluids Discharges up to 2 weeks post lambing
Toxoplasma	6 weeks Infection in early gestation gives reabsorption and apparent barrenness	Feed or forage contaminated with cat faeces No sheep to sheep transmission
Campylobacter	7 days	Carrier sheep Wild life vectors
Salmonella abortus ovis	2 weeks	Carrier sheep
Other salmonella serotypes	1–2 weeks	Food contamination ⎫ Animal protein ⎭ Wildlife vectors Water contamination
Listeria	5–10 days	Poor quality silage High pH, soil contamination
Border disease	Infection <85 days' gestation gives diseased lambs at birth Infection <84 days' gestation gives normal antibody +ve lambs	Virus +ve ⎫ carrier Antibody −ve ⎭ sheep

Guide to diagnosis (see Tables 3.1 and 3.2)

The following points *may* help to give an initial diagnosis, but a final diagnosis *must* rest upon laboratory confirmation, and no possibility should be excluded on macroscopic appearance only. As mentioned previously, beware of mixed or changing causes.

1 Discoloration and necrosis of the cotyledons, oedema or rough thickening of adjacent intercotyledonary tissue, dirty pink or pus-like exudate on placenta surface:

- Suspect *Chlamydia psittaci*.

Note: Q fever (*C. burneti*) is similar in smears, and can be distinguished only on serology, but is much rarer than EAE.

Material	Test	Comments
Placental smear	Modified ZN	Red organisms, singly or in groups, on blue background.
Vaginal discharge	Modified ZN	Take within 24 h of abortion.
Fetal fleece smear	Modified ZN	Organisms sparse, best site is behind ears.
Serology	CFT	>1:32[a] indicates recent infection, use paired samples, or as flock screen.

Note: Where a live but infected lamb is born, pathological change may be limited to a small area of placenta.
Note: Use of EAE vaccine will give positive serology results.

2 *White pinhead-size necrotic foci* present in the cotyledons ('frosted strawberry' appearance), intercotyledonary area normal:

- Suspect toxoplasmosis.

Material	Test	Comments
Fetal pleural fluid	Latex agglutination	1:16 is positive. If LAT is negative, use another test.
Fetal pleural fluid	Indirect fluorescent antibody test (IFAT)	Probably most reliable test.
Fetal pleural fluid	Modified agglutination test	
Fetal pleural fluid	Dye test	
Fetal pleural fluid	ELISA	
Placenta Fetal brain Fetal liver	FAT, histology	

Note: Toxoplasmosis early in pregnancy may cause resorption leading to a large number of barren ewes at lambing time.

3 *Mummified fetuses produced*, with or without normal lambs:

- Check for toxoplasmosis as above.
- Check for border disease, see below.

[a]Titre of 1:32 may be considered to indicate infection in some cases – interpretation varies.

4 Thickened leather-like placenta:

- Check for mycotic abortion (fungal hyphae may be demonstrated in placenta or fetal stomach contents).
- Check for spoilage of homegrown or stored cereals with *Aspergillus fumigatus* or *Fuserium gramminarium.*

5 Characteristic 'hairy shaker' lambs born:

- Check for border disease.

Note: No macroscopic distinguishing features in placenta.

Material	Test	Comments
Placenta, fetal tissues	Virus isolation, IFAT	
Clotted blood from dam and affected lambs	Virus isolation Serology	Presence of antibody only is not diagnostic
Brain and spinal cord	Histopathology	

6 Significant incidence of septicaemia, enteritis and mortality in ewes.

- Suspect salmonellosis.

Material	Test	Comments
Placenta Fetal stomach contents	Smear and culture	Gram-negative organisms
Faeces, intestinal contents, lymph nodes internal organs	Smear and culture	In chronic infections use posterior mesenteric lymph nodes

Note: *S. typhimurium, S. dublin,* usually cause systemic illness. *S. abortus ovis* and *S. montevideo* often cause abortion only.

7 No obvious placental lesions, ewes generally not ill.

- Check for salmonellosis, particularly *S. abortus ovis* (limited to south-west England) and *S. montevideo.* Samples as above.
- Check for *Campylobacter.*

Material	Test	Comments
Placenta and fetal tissue	Smear and culture	
Fetal liver		(Grey necrotic foci sometimes present with *Campylobacter*)

8 Silage fed flock, possibly with neurological signs in ewes or septicaemia in lambs:

● Check for listeriosis.

Material	Test
Fetal tissue	Isolation
Fetal liver	Histology
and placenta	

Note: Abortion due to *Listeria* may occur in absence of neurological disease.

Check quality of silage – soil contamination, high pH, poor fermentation or secondary fermentation all contribute to likelihood of outbreak.

9 Other infectious causes and toxins

There may be sporadic or isolated cases where the following causes may be implicated:

Bacteria such as *Actinomyces* (*Corynebacterium*) *pyogenes, Bacillus licheniformis* (*Br. abortus*).

Tickborne fever – introduction to tick area of unacclimatized pregnant ewes.

Ergotism – infected cereals.

Advice should be sought from the laboratory regarding samples required for investigation.

10 No obvious signs of an infectious agent involved

● Check for recent handling
   e.g. vaccination
         drenching
         excessive use of dogs
         dog worry
● Check condition of ewes
      inadequate feeding
      concurrent disease
      pregnancy toxaemia

Metabolic profiles of at least six ewes may be helpful:
● BHB, plasma protein, urea, glucose.

Note: Micronutrient deficiencies are not thought to be implicated in abortion problems, with the possible exception of vitamin A deficiency.

Fetal overload rarely seems to lead to abortion. In fact, it is surprising how often a pregnancy is maintained in cases of fetal overload or severe undernutrition, putting the life of the ewe at risk, when it would seem that rejection of the fetuses would be the obvious biological solution!

Occasionally, a request for advice is received following an abortion incident when no aborted material is available.

It may be possible to obtain paired sera taken at an interval of 2–3 weeks from affected ewes, providing the first samples are taken soon after abortion, or the clinician may choose to sample those ewes which have aborted and compare with a group which have carried to term with normal viable fetuses. Any results so obtained will need careful interpretation in conjunction with the history of the outbreak.

There is no substitute for early and thorough investigation at the time of the incident, with as much material as possible collected for examination, and this should be stressed to clients in advance of the lambing season via newsletters, practice meetings, etc.

4 Increased incidence of dystocia and vagino-cervical prolapse

Dystocia problems
  Management
  Housing
  Social stress
  Normal litter size
  Fetal oversize
  High litter size
  Failure of cervix to dilate
Cervical/vaginal prolapse
Intestinal prolapse

Perinatal ewe and lamb losses are major components of SORP, and a higher than acceptable incidence of both prolapses and dystocia make important contributions in these areas. Diagnosis is self evident but increasing incidence may bring requests to identify causes. Dystocia increases the perinatal lamb death rate by perhaps 60%. Prolapse of the cervix or vagina places fetal survival at risk by stimulating premature straining, causing changes in intrauterine pressures which jeopardize the integrity of placental circulation. The introduction of infection through a traumatized cervix or an oedematous infected vaginal wall in neglected cases (regrettably common) all too often leads to bacteria gaining entry to the uterine contents and loss of the lambs if not also the ewe.

The clinician must again approach the request for help with a confident knowledge of acceptable proportions of either of these problems for the breed, the management system, and the season. It could be said that zero is the only acceptable incidence but the clinician lives in the real world!

Thus, a flock of Scottish Blackface ewes on normal high hill nutrition, with little social stress, carrying single fetuses of low birth weight will usually experience a very low incidence of dystocia or prolapse. Young Texel ewes on a high plane of nutrition carrying single male lambs have been quoted as requiring manual help for up to 70% of lambings. Surveys of crossbred ewe flocks such as the mule and greyface have revealed a worrying incidence of prolapses reaching 15%, although other flocks have a low incidence.

Superimposed on any 'natural' incidence will be not only the degree of expertise of the shepherd, but also an intangible 'panic' factor which may be the result of 'sympathy', concern for welfare or just plain impatience. The clinician must learn to recognize this when called in to resolve a problem.

It is likely that the clinician will be called in reaction to an unacceptable change for the worse in incidence in an esxtablished flock, but sometimes the call for help may be from a new entrant who has no base line for comparison.

Increase in incidence of dystocia (Figure 4.1)

Normal fetal size, normal litter size

The first check must be for any change in management, primarily intensification, and particularly either a change to a housed system or alterations to that system.

Note: Ewes, if free to do so, will isolate themselves at the onset of the second stage of labour, and then assume dominance in their chosen site for a limited period. If limitations of space prevent this normal behaviour pattern, the parturition process may not proceed smoothly.

- Check overall space per ewe – 1–$1.5\,m^2$ recommended depending on ewe size.
- Check trough space per ewe – 400–500 mm per ewe for concentrates, 200–225 mm for hay or silage feeding *ad libitum*.
- Check age distribution per pen – may be advisable to segregate old and young ewes.
- Check age of high incidence group – social factors may interfere with normal progression of labour.
- Check group size – social stress. Maximum 50 per pen for lowland breeds, 80 for hill breeds.
- Check availability of 'creep' areas – research has shown that parturient ewes will use partially shielded areas if these are provided.
- Check for rams left in groups of housed ewes – aggressive behaviour may lead to physical damage.
- Check experience of shepherd – premature interference can precipitate dystocia where it would not have developed if the ewe had been allowed more time.

Note: This is one of the most difficult areas for the inexperienced to judge, between allowing sufficient time for progress to take place (which can be quite long in primiparous ewes), and not risking the life of the lambs by waiting too long. Recommend attending an Agricultural Training Board lambing course!

Fetal oversize, normal litter size

Note: Relatively minor feto-maternal disproportion may show as high dystocia due to inadequate pelvic inlet area, particularly in young or inexperienced ewes or those of 'suspect' temperament.

- Check feeding in relation to lambing percentage.
- Check if scanning has been carried out. This is of most benefit for flocks lambing at 120–180%, and allows cost-effective feeding of different groups to be carried out.
- Check compatibility of sire breed – choosing the wrong breed can lead to a high degree of feto-maternal disproportion.

- Check lambing spread – later ewes will have had prolonged overfeeding, and are usually less prolific.

Small fetal size, normal litter size

If this problem occurs on a flock basis, the combination must mean that there has been prolonged macro- or micronutrient deprivation, dystocia being either a function of inanition or terminal cachexia. This may be manifest as myometrial inertia associated with calcium deficiency.

- Check body condition score of flock.
- Check for incidence of pregnancy toxaemia.
- Check metabolic profile of representative group of animals (beta hydroxybutyrate, glucose, Ca, P, Mg).

Note: A selenium deficiency in cattle has been shown to be associated with prolonged labour and increased death rate of calves, but there has been no similar picture confirmed in sheep.

Small fetal size, high litter size

A high dystocia rate under these conditions is a function of prolificacy. It must be remembered that prolificacy of itself will increase the incidence of dystocia, partly through the increased risk of malpresentation but also because of a breakdown in the normal dominant/quiescent uterine horn sequence which operates in twinning.

Note: In prolific breeds reproductive output has outstripped the digestive ability to maintain such output. This is partly due to abdominal space limitations, but also to sheer nutrient demand (a ewe with triplets is equal to the demand of a sow with 30+ piglets).

- Check for pregnancy toxaemia induced as a result of fetal demands.
- Check for calcium deficiency.
- Check for abdominal muscle weakness.

Failure of cervix to dilate (ringwomb)

The incidence of failure to dilate varies widely both between flocks and from season to season. Because dystocia inevitably follows, with reduced lamb survival, and because there is always a question mark against future breeding from affected ewes, calls for an explanation will be common.

- Check for prematurity – may be the first evidence of an abortion storm.
- Check for management changes – housing, overcrowding, interference with parturition process.
- Check for malpresentation – no fetus present to complete dilatation.
- Check for calcium deficiency.
- Check for exogenous oestrogens, e.g. home stored corn with fungal contamination (*Fusarium* spp.).

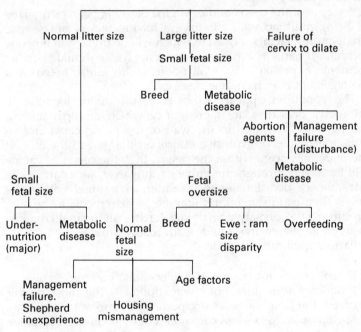

Figure 4.1 Incidence of dystocia

Prolapse of the cervix or vagina/prolapse of the intestines through vaginal rupture

These conditions are grouped as being inextricably linked even though the aetiology is not fully understood. The problem is included in SORP, for although fetal loss is by no means inevitable, except in the case of rupture with prolapse of the intestines where death of ewe and fetuses is extremely rapid, there is a much higher than normal fetal death rate following the occurrence of prolapses. Even if placental integrity is not damaged to a critical point, and live lambs are delivered, the chances of the ewe repeating the condition in future years is so high that it is normal to cull those affected, so adding to culling rate and reducing the true flock output.

Since there is no problem with the diagnosis of this condition, the clinician will only be concerned with aetiology (and treatment), since advice will be required which will reduce losses in future years.

Prolapse of the cervix and/or vagina has long been recognized as being multifactorial, all surveys having picked out several predisposing factors, not all of which will be present in any one incident. It remains a mystery why some flocks should show an incidence of perhaps 15% whilst others with similar breeds and management may have few cases.

The condition appears to be a result of an increase in intrapelvic pressures late in pregnancy, which indirectly activate the pressure receptors in the wall of the pelvic canal and so initiate extremes of expulsive efforts on the part of the ewe. If there are no viscera within the pelvis, then the cervix or vagina will be forced through the vulva. If, however, any part of the intestine, or occasionally the bladder, is trapped within the pelvis then expulsive efforts may be so extreme as to cause a rupture in the dorsal vaginal wall forcing abdominal contents through it. Severe shock and death follow rapidly.

Factors implicated include:

- Breed – check for large pelvic inlets area, e.g. mule.
- Prolificacy (but does not always follow – the most prolific breed, the Cambridge, is not particularly prone to prolapse).
- Multiparous ewes – less common, but by no means unknown in primiparous ewes.
- Bulky feed – sometimes associated with change to silage feeding, or roots.
- Feeding only once daily – splitting both roughage and concentrates into at least two feeds is advisable.
- Fat deposits in abdomen or pelvis – overfatness, particularly in young ewes.
- Steep slope in field allowing abdominal contents to 'drift' into pelvis during sleep or cudding (heavily pregnant ewes always stand or lie facing uphill which eases some of the pressure on the thorax).

- Reduced perineal support – short docking may reduce muscular support of posterior vagina and vulva. Short docking is illegal.
- Chronic cough (rather unlikely on flock basis).
- Reduced calcium concentrations have been implicated, but whether as a primary cause or secondary to stress is not clear.

The clinician is left, therefore, with a detailed history taking to establish which factor or combination of factors is the cause of any one incident. Usually many will be able to be eliminated, but is what is left the answer? At the end of the investigation we may be left unable to identify the exact cause, but breed and strain do have a big effect, and there is probably a hereditary component. There seems to be little doubt that the incidence is reaching worrying proportions in some flocks.

5 Male infertility

Poor libido
Group infertility
Individual infertility
Ram examination
Semen collection and examination

Routine examination of the ram before the breeding season begins is now a recognized procedure in the sheep industry, but even so, only a minority of animals actually are examined. Requests are commonly made for the examination of individual rams of suspect fertility, or for assistance in flocks experiencing apparent difficulties getting ewes in lamb, and it is with these aspects that this text is concerned. Surveys have suggested that some 10% of rams are likely to be infertile, with a further 30% being of suspect fertility.

The UK is generally regarded as being free of major genital infections such as *Brucella ovis*, genital actinobacillosis and scrotal mange, which are serious problems in some parts of the world. In the absence of these major infectious conditions, a fertility problem on any particular unit is likely to be made up of a number of individual cases of differing aetiology.

Note: *Histophilus ovis* infection, which occurs in a number of other countries, was isolated from rams with epididymitis in the UK in 1985, and may ultimately prove to be more of a problem than is presently recognized.

Incidents involving whole groups of rams

Infections of the external genitalia of both ewes and rams occasionally occur around mating time, but do *not* generally cause infertility. Mycoplasmas and ureaplasms have been isolated from some of these cases of balanoposthitis and vulvovaginitis but their significance is not clear.

- Check also for orf virus.
- Check for short tail docking in ewes – fly nuisance may be significant.
- If sponges used, check hygiene and technique.

Note: In the immediate pre-mating period, the male group often indulges in mounting behaviour. This frequently results in insertion of the penis into the rectum of other rams, leading to contamination with faeces – it is not known whether this can act as a source of infection.

Individual male infertility

Detection and identification of an infertile male will be no problem in small flocks or pedigree flocks where a single male is used. In larger flocks, without routine examination of all rams, detection of an infertile male will often be difficult, as the rams are usually run in groups with large numbers of ewes. The rams may well be of differing ages and will always be of varying dominance, aggression and libido. In addition, it is normal for the ewe to 'seek out' the ram, and the female group will have an established order of dominance.

A combination of these two patterns can give rise to quite complex social interactions, which may mask not only the true fertility rate, but may also hinder the search for an infertile animal. As an example, if a particular male is extremely aggressive he may spend the whole period preventing access by other rams in the group to females in oestrus, but may not himself mate, either through exhaustion or by constantly defending the ewe group from other males. Conversely, an older dominant ewe may 'appropriate' the male for such a long period that other ewes remain unmated.

Although it has been established that trained rams are capable of producing fertile semen throughout the year, in the field there is undoubtedly a strong photoperiodic effect in the male as well as the female. Finn, Friesland and Milksheep rams will be active very early in the breeding season, and the Suffolk soon after. In contrast, the Texel is notoriously late (fully fertile rams may show little interest until late September).

Just as the early onset of puberty in the female and prolificacy appear to have a strong correlation, so in the male early puberty is linked to the seasonal duration of active sexual drive. In addition, there is a correlation between large testicle size in relation to body weight and the early onset of puberty.

Where a flock fertility problem exists, the investigation of the male role in this will be in two stages:
(1) Establishing the validity and nature of the problem.
(2) Diagnosis of the cause by observation of behaviour and clinical examination.

Requests may be made to examine a ram at the end of the lambing season, for example, if rams of different breeds were used and few offspring of one were born. This is *not* a suitable time to make an accurate assessment, and examination should be delayed until nearer the normal mating season.

Apparent sexual inactivity

• Check ewes are not already in lamb.

Before any detailed investigations of the ram, establish if the complaint is valid. *The most common cause of non-mating is pregnancy.* This should be detectable from about 30 days with a Doppler pregnancy detector, and 50 days with a scanner. If vasectomized rams have been used in the flock, check these for time of surgery in relation to exposure to ewes (a minimum of 2 weeks should be allowed), or misidentification of teaser rams.

- Check for body condition – if ram is too thin, suspect nutrition or concurrent disease (see chapter 12 on adult weight loss).
- If ram is too fat, check for overfeeding.
- Newly purchased high value rams may show temporary infertility due to sudden change in environment and nutrition.
- If ram is in good body condition (3.5–4.5 body score), check for breed or season incompatibility.
- Check for immaturity – testicle size.
- Check if young inexperienced ram is with inexperienced females – may be better with older ewes.
- Check if young ram was reared in all-male group – may be shy when put with group of females.

If the above factors are eliminated, the clinician must establish whether the ram really has poor libido, or if he is incapable of demonstrating interest because of other disease factors, in particular interference with mobility.

- Check for footrot, foot abscess, arthritis, lumbar pain.
- Check for other concurrent disease – parasites, pulmonary or cardiac disease.

Low libido

This may be the transitional phase to or from the last section.

- Check as above.
- Check for onset of exhaustion – if libido was normal earlier in breeding season, may be overwork. Ram:ewe ratio recommended is 1:25 for ram lamb and 1:40 or 50 for mature ram, except in synchronized flocks (see chapter 2).
- Check for small testicle size.

Note: Serving capacity can be correlated with testicle size. Tests for serving capacity have been established in New Zealand and Australia, but are not in common use here because of possible welfare problems.

Note: An apparent lack of sexual activity in the daytime does not preclude full activity during darkness. Raddle or harnesses should be used to obtain firm evidence.

Normal libido, little mounting activity

- Check for pregnancy.
- Check for pain focus in those structures most involved in the mounting process – hindlimb lameness, poor hindlimb conformation, lumbar or pelvic pain.
- Check for painful lesion of penis or prepuce.

Normal libido, normal mounting, failure to mate

Note: The clinician must be able to differentiate between mounting and full mounting with intromission and thrusting during ejaculation.

- Check for inexperience – age and previous use.
- Check ability to extrude penis fully.
- Check for abnormality of the penis, either anatomical or traumatic, e.g. deviation.

Normal libido, normal mating behaviour, high return rate

Before blaming the ram, the clinician should be satisfied that there are no adverse factors affecting the fertility of the ewes (see chapter 2). In particular:

- Check ewe:ram ratio.
- Check that synchronization problems are not involved.
- Check that expectations are not too great at either end of normal breeding season.
- Check for recent illness in ram – pyrexia can induce temporary infertility.

A full clinical examination of the ram should then be carried out. This will be essentially the same examination as that carried out in the pre-breeding check, but will always require the collection and examination of a semen sample unless gross lesions accounting for the fertility problem are detected.

Routine for the clinical examination of a ram

General examination (see Table 5.1 and Figure 5.1):

- Check the general health and conformation.
  Condition score
  Head, mouth, eyes
  Legs, feet, stance, gait
- Check for evidence of gross lesions of the genitalia.

With ram in the standing position check:

- Number of testicles
- Size and symmetry of testicles
- Shape of testicles – ovoid not cylindrical
- Presence and size of head and tail of epididymis
- Mobility of testicles within scrotum
- Obvious palpable abnormalities
- Absence of inguinal herniation
- Absence of heavy wool cover on scrotum

Note: Full spermatogenesis is dependent upon the testicles being maintained at several degrees below body temperature. Heavy wool cover will interfere with this mechanism, but after shearing it will take 6–8 weeks to return to normal function, as this is the length of time required for maturation of sperm.

Approximate testicular dimensions in normal rams
Adult ram, scrotal diameter, 36 cm
Testicle length, 10–11 cm
Testicle diameter, 7–8 cm
Epididymis diameter, 3.5–4 cm

These figures are those which could be expected in mature rams of medium/large breeds, at the beginning of the breeding season. Ram lambs and adults of small breeds will show slightly smaller dimensions. Out of the breeding season, these measurements may be considerably reduced, and an opinion on fertility should not be given unless gross abnormalities are present.

With ram in upright sitting position check:

- Extent of inguinal 'blush' inside thighs (marked erythema of skin) indicating testosterone surge.
- Scrotal skin for thickening or scarring (including vasectomy scars).
- Testicles for evidence of asymmetry in texture.
- Testicular size in relation to breed, maturity, time of year.

Table 5.1 Ram examination check list

Owner
Address
Date
Ram ear number
Breed
Age
Condition score
Teeth
Feet and legs
Other remarks on general condition

Scrotum	diameter		
	abnormalities		
Testicles	length	R	L
	diameter	R	L
	resilience	R	L
	abnormalities	R	L
Epididymis	tail diameter	R	L
	resilience	R	L
	abnormalities	R	L

Prepuce
Penis and appendage

Semen	volume	colour
	density	motility
	live:dead ratio	
	abnormalities	

Verdict

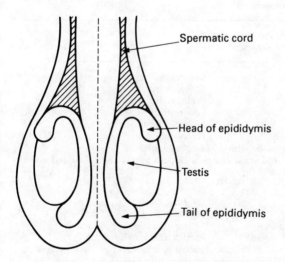

Figure 5.1 Scrotal anatomy

- Testicular resilience: 25–30% deformation is normal, 40% is too soft, <20% is too hard – scar tissue.
- Developmental abnormality, e.g. spermatocele.
- Epididymis for presence and normality of head and tail, or epididymitis.
- Prepuce for evidence of trauma or infection.
- Preputial orifice for trauma or infection.

Extrude penis and check for:
- Full extrusion, normal length
- Injury or anatomical defects
- Urethral fistula
- Presence of appendage

Note: The function of the appendage is almost certainly to spray semen at increased pressure over the cervix. Total absence without subsequent scar tissue is probably of less significance than a partial absence which may cause 'misdirection' of the ejaculate.

Table 5.2 Hereditary defects in the ram

Cryptorchid
Testicular hypoplasia
Testicular aplasia
Inguinal hernia
Entropion
Poor incisor tooth apposition

Table 5.2 Appearance of semen

Sperm density	Comment
Watery <0.5 × 10^9/ml	Probably infertile
Cloudy 0.5–1 × 10^9/ml	Probably infertile
Milky 1–3 × 10^9/ml	Low fertility
Creamy 3–4 × 10^9/ml	Probably fertile
Thick creamy >4 × 10^9/ml	Probably fertile

Accurate counts can be made with a haemocytometer
Heavily worked rams could show semen with poor appearance. Rest and retest after 1–2 weeks

Motility	Comment
None	Infertile, dead
Slow wave motion	Low fertility <50% activity
Distinct waves with motion	Probably fertile 70–80% activity
Dark waves with rapid motion	Ideal >80% activity

*Beware of cold shock which will affect motility. If semen has cooled warm gently and re-examine. This may revive sperm if cold shock was not severe

If no evidence of gross pathology is detected, then the clinician must proceed to a full semen examination. In contrast to the situation when routine pre-service examinations are carried out, when there is some question as to the necessity to ejaculate a ram which appears physically normal, there is an obligation to carry out not only ejaculation but also a full examination, including staining and evaluation of the semen sample (see Table 5.3).

Note: When collecting a semen sample, great care should be taken to avoid cold shock which will give a false impression of the quality of the sample.

Equipment required for semen collection and examination

Microscope with ×40, ×100 and oil immersion lenses.
Plate warmer or flat-sided bottle filled with water at body temperature.
Clean slides.
5% nigrosin/eosin stain (freshly prepared if possible).
Ram ejaculator, batteries, lubricant.
Collection tubes and funnel or small polythene bags.
Waterproof marker pen.
Record sheet.

Restraint of ram during collection

Collection may be carried out with the ram either standing, or restrained in lateral recumbency, according to personal preference. If, when using the electro-ejaculator, no sample is obtained after three stimulations of approximately 4 seconds each, the ram should be rested for 30 min before trying again. Semen should be collected into a warmed container and immediately transferred to a warm environment to avoid cold shock.

● Check semen quantity.
● Check semen density – creamy, watery, milky, marbled, clotted, haemorrhagic.
● Check motility (low power) – dense waves, waves forming and dissolving; quivering may indicate urine contamination.

Make stained smear with fresh nigrosin/eosin (1 drop semen to 3–5 drops stain), examine with oil immersion lens:

- Check sperm density.
- Check live:dead ratio (dead sperm stain pink, live sperm repel stain and are colourless).
- Check normal:abnormal ratio.

Characteristics of normal semen

Volume – 0.5–2 ml.
Density – thick, creamy colour.
Motility – distinct or fast swirling wave motion.
Dead or abnormal sperm – <20%.
Note: Some coiled or reflected tails are generally thought not to be of significance – probably an artifact due to technique of staining.

It is only at this stage that a verdict on the likely cause of subfertility in the individual ram can be attempted.

Note: No ram should be considered as infertile on the basis of a single unsatisfactory semen examination, in the absence of gross pathological change. Spermatogenesis and libido may fluctuate. There is also a time delay of some 6–8 weeks between the end of any interference with full sperm production and the appearance of a normal sample. Except in the presence of gross abnormalities, an opinion should not be passed on a ram outside the normal breeding season.

In the end, the only true evidence of fertility is pregnancy.

6 Periparturient ewe losses

Before parturition
During parturition
Post parturition
Postmortem examination

It is estimated that some 4–6% of ewes die annually, perhaps up to 10% in hill units, and that of these about three-quarters are lost at or near lambing. These losses will rarely be 'sudden deaths', many of the ewes having exhibited symptoms of illness and probably having received treatment of some kind. Many deaths are undoubtedly related to mismanagement of factors such as prolapses, or obstetrical interferences, but it is likely to be the exceptional shepherd who volunteers responsibility for a death by admitting ineptitude. However, deaths do occur at this time in spite of the best endeavours of conscientious and skilled shepherd care, but a death rate in large units of above 2% (except in difficult environmental conditions) should give rise to concern.

This chapter deals specifically with losses related to pregnancy and parturition, and in particular with the flock which exhibits an unacceptable rise in losses. Further relevant information may be found in chapter 22 on sudden death and in Appendix 1 on postmortem examination.

In any investigation of a flock with an unacceptably high periparturient ewe loss the following facts need to be established:

● The history of the incident.
● Incidence of losses in relation to previous seasons.
● Timing of losses in relation to parturition.
● Body condition of affected ewes and rest of group.
● Any signs observed.
● Any treatments given and their efficacy.
● Vaccination history of the flock.

In particular the following factors should be checked out (see also Table 6.1 and Figure 6.1).

If losses are before lambing period

● Check how far from lambing.
● Check body condition and nutrition.
● Check for evidence of impending abortion – vaginal discharge. (See chapter 3.)
● Check for scouring – possible salmonellosis.
● Check for evidence of recumbency – excoriation of lower limbs, trauma to eye area, hypostatic congestion. This may indicate metabolic disease (calcium deficiency or pregnancy toxaemia).

Table 6.1 Aids to diagnosis in periparturient ewe losses

	Gross pathology	*Biochemistry*	*Microbiology*
Pregnancy toxaemia	Fatty liver Fetal overload Poor fat reserves or overfat	Ketones in urine, reduced plasma glucose, raised BHB	–
Hypocalcaemia	None	Ca, P and Mg in aqueous humour or CSF	–
Septicaemia	Petechiae, fluid in serous cavities		Heart blood, liver, lung, spleen, for culture
Clostridial disease	Haemorrhage and gas in affected area, especially perineum		Tissue for IFAT
Abortion		← See chapter 3 →	

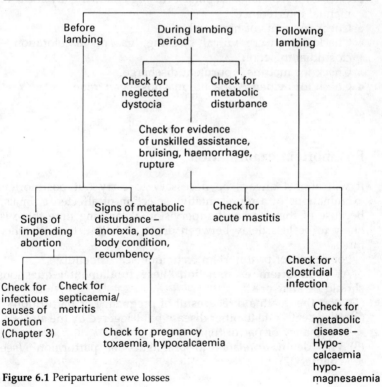

Figure 6.1 Periparturient ewe losses

Note: Aqueous humour is a useful sampling fluid, as concentrations of minerals and metabolites are stable for up to 48 h.

If losses are during lambing period

- Check as above *plus* . . .
- Check if parturition has commenced – evidence of fetal fluids, fetal parts, or placenta.
- Check skill of shepherd, students or other helpers.
- Check for external evidence of bruising or trauma of vulval area, haemorrhage.
- Check for concurrent abortion problem.
- Check for neglected cervical or vaginal prolapse.
- Check for prolapsed intestines.

If losses occur after lambing

- Check for vulval or vaginal bruising following dystocia or manual interference.
- Check for signs of haemorrhage.
- Check for severe vulval swelling, gas or discoloration – clostridial infection.
- Check for metritis – purulent discharge.
- Check for evidence of acute mastitis – gangrene.

Postmortem examination

It will almost always be necessary to carry out postmortem examinations of a representative selection of affected animals. Because of the degree of supervision at lambing time there is likely to be less delay between death and PME than at other times.

For details of postmortem technique see Appendix 1.

At postmortem examination these fundamental questions should be answered:

(1) Was the death a direct result of pregnancy or parturition?
(2) Was death due to other disease but triggered by the stress of pregnancy or parturition?
(3) Was death unrelated to pregnancy or parturition? (see chapter 22)

Particular points to note during the postmortem examination

Death before commencement of parturition (cervix closed)

- Check for poor nutrition – condition, fat deposits.
- Check for nutrition-related disease – pregnancy toxaemia (fatty liver, urine sample for ketones).
- Check for metabolic disease – calcium deficiency (sample aqueous humour).
- Check the placenta for evidence of separation.
- Check for placentitis – impending abortion.
- Check the fetus for time of death in relation to maternal death.
- Check for disease unrelated to pregnancy, e.g. pasteurellosis.

Death during parturition (cervix partly or completely open)

- Check for dystocia – ringwomb, malpresentation.

Note: If the cervix is patent, fetal autolysis is very rapid within the uterus (death, emphysema and disintegration may take as little as 48 h).

- Check for manual interference – bruising, haemorrhage, trauma.
- Check for impending abortion, placentitis, mummification.
- Check for signs of septicaemia.
- Check for catastrophe – torsion of uterus, rupture.
- Check for other disease unrelated to parturition.

Death after parturition completed

- Check for manual interference – bruising, trauma, haemorrhage, uterine rupture.
- Check for retained placenta, or metritis.

Note: Placental separation normally occurs very rapidly, and in contrast to the cow, retention is rare.

- Check for clostridial infection – rapid decomposition, gas in tissues.
- Check for choking on fetal membranes.
- Check for metabolic disease – calcium or magnesium deficiency (aqueous humour sample).
- Check for acute mastitis.

Note: Particular care must be taken in the interpretation of any bacteriological results of material taken from the uterus if parturition has started or been completed, since bacteria will have been introduced in any manual interference.

7 Mastitis, udder and teat lesions

Organisms implicated
Udder problems at lambing
Insufficient colostrum production
Supply/demand imbalance
Udder problems during lactation
Udder problems after weaning/at culling
Teat lesions
Dairy sheep flocks

Mastitis is an important cause of premature culling, and estimates of a 5–10% annual culling rate for this reason have been suggested. In a slaughterhouse survey of culled ewes, 50% were found to have udder abnormalities.

Initially, it would appear that the diagnosis of mastitis in the ewe is so self evident that it does not require any amplification. However, the advent of sheep milk production as a method of diversification, where the pattern of mastitis resembles that in the dairy cow, and the entry of many new owners into the sheep industry have altered this situation.

In flocks other than dairy sheep, cases of mastitis are usually presented to the veterinarian at a much later stage in the disease process than is the case with dairy cattle, because there is no day-to-day inspection of the udder. Thus a diagnosis will have been made and the request will be for assistance in treatment. The clinician will be concerned with changes in incidence, the causes of such change, and future prevention rather than the diagnosis of the presence or absence of overt disease.

In some cases, particularly where the owner is inexperienced, a sheep with acute mastitis may be presented as a case of lameness, since often the first sign of acute mastitis is dragging of the hind leg on the affected side. It is essential, therefore, that the clinician check the udder if the patient is near to lambing, lactating or in the immediate post-weaning period. In addition, the presence of udder or teat lesions should always be suspected if lambs appear constantly hungry, or if the ewe does not stand to allow hungry lambs to suck.

Non-dairy flocks

Bacteriological tests are always necessary to determine the cause of mastitis cases, since there are no clinically distinguishing features.

The following organisms have been implicated most common-ly:

Pasteurella haemolytica
Staphylococcus aureus
Streptococcus spp.
E. coli
Actinomyces (Corynebacterium) pyogenes.

Mixed infections involving P. haemolytica or Staph. aureus are also common.

Note: Most of these organisms are normal commensal bacteria. *P. haemolytica* is thought to be transferred from the pharynx of the lamb to the teat of the ewe. Organisms then presumably gain entry into the udder via the teat canal, because of some loss of the defensive integrity of the teat sphincter and canal. Teat and udder lesions are, therefore, closely linked to the incidence of mastitis.

The condition is most commonly seen at four stages in the production cycle (see Table 7.1).

(1) At or near lambing (often the results of an earlier infection which only becomes apparent at this time).
(2) At 4–8 weeks of lactation.
(3) After weaning.
(4) At the culling examination.

Table 7.1 Mastitis

Stage of lactation	Predisposing factors
Periparturient	Weaning policy Inadequate culling examination
Full lactation	Supply/demand imbalance Large litters Inadequate nutrition Failure to provide lamb creeps Orf infection Teat lesions Udder exposure – winter shearing, short docking, excessive crutching, lack of shelter
Mid/late lactation	Supply/demand imbalance Marketing policy – removal of one of twins
Post-weaning/culling exam	Weaning policy – removal of one lamb only, no reduced inputs to discourage lactation No use of dry ewe therapy

Udder problems at lambing

Factors such as poor teat conformation, injury, or the inability of the lamb to suck may predispose to mastitis if the udder is not emptied.

If individual ewes have congested udders, or lambs are hungry:

- Check if clinical mastitis is present.
- Check teat canal for patency.
- Wax plug may block teat (this is normal, and is usually removed when the lambs first suck).
- Occlusion of the canal with a 'fibrous' cord indicates infection during a previous lactation.
- Absence of canal (congenital).
- Inverted teats (congenital).
- Shearing injury (partial or complete removal of teat).
- Check teat/udder conformation – 'bottle tits'.
- Check lamb viability – can it suck?

If many ewes have insufficient colostrum at lambing:
- Check ewe condition and feeding in late pregnancy.
- *Leptospira interrogans var. hardjo* infection has been reported as a cause of lack of milk in groups of otherwise apparently healthy ewes.
    If suspected take blood and milk samples for culture at time of milk lack.
    Positive serology is *not* necessarily evidence of disease as this is apparently quite widespread.

Udder problems at 4–8 weeks into lactation period

- Check for insufficient milk to supply demands of lambs.

In the case of prolific ewes suckling multiples, especially triplets, the lambs may make constant demands upon the ewe for milk. This is particularly seen if no special arrangements have been made to manage them separately as far as ewe nutrition and provision of lamb creeps are concerned. Competition for teats often leads to teat damage with the formation of painful thickened plaques on the medial surface of the teats, in the position at which the incisor teeth of the lambs contact the teats. Ewes usually refuse to allow the lambs to suck, and mastitis is a common sequel.

- Check for staphylococcal and/or *Pasteurella* infection of teats.
- Check for orf lesions. These may begin on the lambs' mouths and be transferred to the teats or vice versa. Dry scabs should be submitted for confirmation by electron microscopy.
- Check for orf vaccination of ewes too close to lambing – transfer of vaccine virus via lambs to teats (minimum recommended time between ewe vaccination and lambing is 8 weeks).

- Check for use of orf vaccine in lambs without prior ewe vaccination.
- Check for winter shearing, or excessive crutching. There is a suggestion that these practices predispose to mastitis because of chilling of the udder. There is also a suggestion of breed susceptibility, e.g. mule.
- Check for oversupply of milk.

This period coincides with a change from primarily 'milk nutrition' in the lamb, to primarily 'grass based' nutrition. In the case of ewe breeds with a high lactation potential on high planes of nutrition, supply and demand for milk will rapidly become out of balance. The resultant back pressure will act as a potential cause of udder inflammation and infection as has been established for many years in the dairy cow.

Udder problems after weaning

Many of these infections are subclinical during the suckling phase and only become apparent after weaning. Sudden removal of the lambs, with a build up of milk in the udder, allows the infection to become clinically apparent. There is the common danger that many such infections will not be identified until the culling inspection, by which time permanent damage to udder function will have occurred.

- Check weaning technique – removal of one of twins (e.g. early prime lamb for slaughter) may result in one side of the udder becoming distended. Unless careful watch can be kept on the udder it may be better management to wean both lambs simultaneously.
- Check for feeding after weaning – short period on minimal inputs, e.g. straw, may be necessary to rapidly terminate lactation.
- Check for healed teat lesions, over-sucking, orf.
- Check if any use of dry ewe therapy.

Udder problems at the culling inspection

These infections are those described in the previous paragraph, i.e. which occurred at weaning, but were not noticed at that time, since concurrent systemic disease is rare. The clinician is not likely to be called in to identify the presence of such lesions, but only requested to find reasons for high or changed incidence. Weaning management is likely to be implicated.

Dairy sheep flocks

It is becoming apparent that mastitis occurs in the dairy sheep flock in very similar patterns to those which exist in the dairy cattle industry. Presumably the stresses of machine milking, with all the risks of damage to the integrity of the teat and sphincter, are very similar.

The changes to the udder are not usually as severe as those in the ewe suckling her lamb, although gangrenous mastitis can occur. This is not primarily due to differing infections, but because the sheep milker has the same frequent opportunities as the cow milker to observe changes in the udder, and therefore to initiate treatment, and control. In addition, the practice of preventive therapy is much more justified in this type of enterprise.

When called to the 'milking' flock the clinician will have a large body of experience to apply to the control of the problem. Diagnosis and treatment should be carried out as for the dairy cow, for the dairy sheep is effectively 'a cow with wool' rather than a sheep which happens to give a lot of milk.

The investigation will include:

- Assessment of parlour and dairy hygiene.
- Use of udder washes and disposable teat cloths.
- Milking routine.
- Teat dipping.
- Milking machine maintenance.

The present state of knowledge of sheep milking machine technology is still in the developmental stage, so optimum vacuum and pulsation rates are not well established. Reference should be made to the milking machine manufacturer for further advice.

8 Perinatal lamb losses

Acceptable/unacceptable rates of loss
Lamb postmortem examination routine
Antepartum deaths
Intrapartum deaths
  Managemental
  Infections

The success or failure of a flock depends to a large extent on its performance around lambing time. Attention has already been drawn to the importance of periparturient ewe losses, which form a large proportion of the estimated 10% total annual ewe losses. Although the lambing percentage for the UK as a whole is approximately 125%, it is disturbing but true that the net output is less than 100%, and analysis of flock outputs has shown that as many as 5 million lambs which have reached full term fail to reach the point of sale. The figures for ewe and lamb losses taken together give an alarming overall annual death rate of about 17% of the total sheep population.

Clearly, then, the efficient sheep keeper experiencing significant losses will be concerned with the cause and will require answers from an advisor within a very short time scale, i.e. within *this* lambing season.

Numerous surveys of lamb losses have indicated that some 90% of these occur perinatally. Losses in individual flocks vary widely depending on husbandry, weather, shepherd skill, etc., but may exceed 25% of those born. Indeed, some flock owners may be unable to give an accurate figure, preferring to remain in ignorant bliss! There will be the added complication that analysis of losses has concluded that 'whilst ewe losses are due to disease, lamb losses are due to management' which, taken with the fatalism of some older traditional shepherds that 'you are always going to lose some lambs' may lead to communication difficulties.

Institution of some form of record keeping must, therefore, be a priority in any such flock, but it must be realized that whilst it is easy for the clinician to insist on full records from the security of a warm surgery, it is not so simple for the shepherd to record in detail the results of a very difficult lambing – a sick ewe, three stinking lambs, and six more sheep 'waiting'!

What then are the normally expected or acceptable losses?

- Zero should be that which is acceptable.
- Less than 5% should be that which is expected.

In reality, losses of more than 10% are 'normal' even in lowland conditions, whilst on the high hill the figure may reach several times higher.

The clinician must be aware of the pattern of loss during the whole perinatal period if valid advice is to be given.

Losses occur in two phases:
(1) lambs born dead are often quoted as 8–10%,
(2) lambs dying in the first 72 h are often quoted as 10–12%.

In fact, these figures contain great untruths. If lambing is carried out under a regime of total shepherding, i.e. 24-h supervision, then the truly 'born dead' figure is often extremely low (2–3%), showing that, in all probability, in less supervised flocks many of those classed as 'born dead' were actually alive but failed to live because no-one was present to revive them. If the same management pressure is applied within the next 72 h, then the losses during this time are reduced to 1–2%.

Thus the difference between these 'unavoidable' deaths and the generally accepted rates quoted above could be classed as 'avoidable' deaths.

(Whether it is good policy to adopt the 'save everything' attitude, and perhaps perpetuate inherited characteristics such as poor mothering ability, is another matter!)

So we are left with the fact that lamb losses *are* essentially a result of failures in management. MLC figures comparing losses in top third performing flocks with those in average and bottom third performing flocks confirm that improvements are achievable, with number of lambs reared being responsible for 20% of their superiority. It must be recognized, however, that even in well managed flocks lambing out of doors, sudden adverse weather conditions can have a marked influence on these figures in spite of the best efforts of the shepherd.

It is against this difficult background that the clinician must operate, and will require in addition to good clinical skills, top quality communication abilities if conclusions are to be accepted and applied by both owner and shepherd.

Flock investigation (Figure 8.1)

Attempts should be made to categorize the losses into antepartum (e.g. abortion agents), intrapartum (dystocia), or postpartum. By far the most important cause in this last category, accounting for some 30–50%, is hypothermia (starvation and/or chilling) which is often the result of the dystocia–mismothering–exposure–starvation sequence.

In obtaining a history and carrying out a general examination of the flock, the following points will be of particular relevance:

- breed
- normal litter size and lamb weights
- hardiness
- ewe nutrition particularly in last 8 weeks of pregnancy

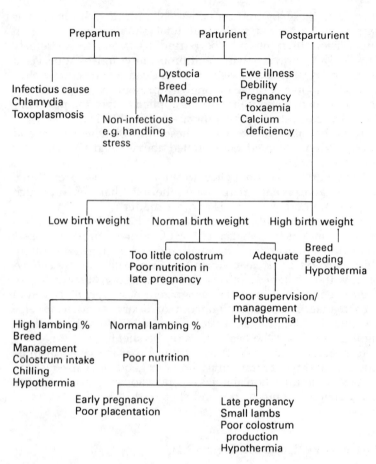

Figure 8.1 Investigation of periparturient lamb losses

- ewe condition scores
- vaccination history
- age group of ewes from which losses are occurring, e.g. young, old, thin, fat
- any signs of infectious agents operating in ewes, e.g. abortions, or lambs, e.g. enteritis
- colostrum production by ewes, i.e. udder development, teat function
- lamb management immediately after birth
- routine for checking colostrum intake

- use of stomach tube
- provision of colostrum bank (species used?)
- method of defrosting and heating colostrum (overheating will denature IgG)
- hygiene in lambing pens
- navel hygiene
- timing of castration and docking if done
- use of individual lambing pens (bonding)
- management of multiples especially triplets, quads, etc.
- provision of heat lamps or warming boxes
- outdoor management, availability of shelter.

Postmortem examination

In any investigation of unacceptable lamb losses, it is essential that as much postmortem material as possible is examined. Do not rely on the findings in only a small number of carcases as there may well be a multiplicity of causes of death.

Although the following list seems alarmingly long, the technique of postmortem examination in young lambs is usually simple and quick to carry out. In combination with laboratory help where necessary, it will usually allow the clinician to identify the main stages and area(s) of loss. Examination should be carried out in a logical manner so that shortcuts are not taken which may lead to inaccurate diagnosis. Where infectious conditions are suspected, e.g. neonatal septicaemia or enteritis, samples should be selected as the postmortem examination proceeds. The most useful samples will be liver, spleen, lung, heart blood; in addition, intestinal contents plus mesenteric lymph node for enteritis, joint fluid in polyarthritis, brain for swayback and border disease.

Checklist for PME of young lamb

Single/twin/triplet/quad
Fullterm/premature
Weight – normal/underweight/excessively large
Fresh/decomposing/mummified
Fleece dry/wet – fetal fluid/meconium staining/rain-soaked
Fleece type – normal/premature/excessively hairy
Predator damage – after/before death (signs of haemorrhage)
Eyes – normal/sunken (dehydration)

Cornea – clear/opaque
Mouth – clean/wet/congenital deformity/trauma/orf
Navel – wet/dry/antibiotic spray or iodine applied/thickened/
    infected
Feet – walked/not walked (foot membranes present)
Anal region – meconium/orange colostral/scour/blood
Subcutaneous oedema – dystocia (part of body?)/hypothermia
    (extremities, yellow colour)
Muscles – colour/dryness/wasting
Blood – normal/watery
Abdominal cavity – clear fluid (<1 ml is normal)/fibrin/blood
Umbilical arteries – end straight/end tapered/clot
Bladder ligament – normal/oedema/fibrin/pus
Abomasum – milk clot/liquid milk/saliva/gas/wool/empty
Intestines – food present/absent/hyperaemia/gas/torsion (small
    undigested clots in colon indicate alimentary problem)
Food absorption – good/poor/absent (mesenteric lacteals should
    be white up to or beyond mesenteric lymph nodes if
    absorption is good)
Meconium/faeces – present/absent/imperforate anus
Liver – haemorrhage/rupture/abscesses
Kidneys – normal/autolysed/enlarged/pale (nephrosis)
Perirenal fat – normal/metabolized (gelatinous, pink)
Ribs – fractures
Thorax – clear fluid/fibrin/haemorrhage
Lungs – uninflated (sinks in water)/partially inflated/fully
    inflated (floats in water)/pneumonia
Pleural cavity – fluid (<1 ml normal)/pleurisy
Pericardium – fluid/fibrin/fat present/metabolized
Heart – congenital defects
Epicardial fat – present/metabolized
Joints – normal/enlarged
Joint fluid – absent/clear/cloudy/pus
Bone marrow – red/pale
Brain – haemorrhage/cavitation/congenital deformity

Note: Brown fat stores are metabolized in a set order. It is thus
possible to assess the degree of starvation. Pericardial fat is used
first, followed by that in the coronary groove, around the left
coronary artery and finally the renal fat. If these last two sites
are metabolized (indicated by gelatinous pinky material),
starvation is definitely indicated.

As a result of this examination it should be possible to place
the death in one of the following categories (see Table 8.1).

Table 8.1 Time of death in common diseases in lambs

Prepartum	Maternal disease, e.g. pregnancy toxaemia, hypocalcaemia Placental insufficiency – fetal overload Abortion – infectious agents
Partum	Dystocia Maternal disease, e.g. pregnancy toxaemia, hypocalcaemia
Postpartum	At birth – Parturient trauma

At birth – Parturient trauma
             Congenital disease — swayback, border disease,
                              cerebellar hypoplasia,
                              nutritional myopathy
Hours — Failure to suck – Hypothermia
          Exposure
          Mismothering
Days 1 — Watery mouth
          Hypothermia
    2 — Lamb dysentery
          Enteritis (*E. coli, Rotavirus*)
          Neonatal polyarthritis
          Navel ill
    3 — Liver abscess
    4 — Spinal abscess
    7 —   Orf

Any time: accident – trauma – predator

	Features
Antepartum	
dead a long time	Mummification, autolysis, collapse of eyeball.
recently dead	No thrombus in umbilical artery, square end to artery.
Intrapartum	
early in parturition	No thrombus in umbilical artery, tapered end to artery, renal autolysis.
late in parturition	No thrombus in umbilical artery, tapered end, no renal autolysis, localized oedema.
Postpartum	
in first few minutes	Thrombus at end of umbilical artery, lungs uninflated.
in first few hours	Lungs inflated, hoof membrane present but may be beginning to separate, navel cord wet.
lived a few days	Hooves hardened, navel shrivelled.

Guide to cause of death (see also Table 8.2)

Antepartum deaths

Mummification, autolysis, collapse of eyeball, haemoglobin staining all indicate dead a long time.

- Check for *Toxoplasma*, border disease. See chapter 3.

Renal autolysis, but little autolysis of rest of body, some corneal opacity, wool loosening, square end to umbilical artery with no thrombus (or sometimes thrombus whole way along) indicate dead only a few days prepartum:

- Check for infectious cause, e.g. *Chlamydia*. See chapter 3.
- Check for fetal overload, placental insufficiency.
- Check for recent handling, dog worry, etc.
- Check for maternal disease – pregnancy toxaemia, calcium deficiency, vaginal prolapse.

Table 8.2 Predisposing factors in lamb deaths

Problem	Result
Abortion	Premature low birthweight lambs
Poor ewe body condition	Low birthweight lambs, poor colostrum supply
Ewe age	Young – inexperienced mothers
	Old – poor colostrum supply
Ewe disease	Poor maternal ability
	Poor colostrum supply
Litter size	Inadequate colostrum for all lambs
Birth weight	High – dystocia
	Low – hypothermia
Dystocia	Hypoxaemia ⎤ Poor temperature
	Subcranial haemorrhage ⎦ regulation
Housing	Reduces hypothermia risk
	Increases infection risk
Weather	Cold, wind, rain, snow increase
	Hypothermia risk

Intrapartum deaths

Pointed end to umbilical artery, no thrombus, renal autolysis, little localized oedema indicate death early in parturition.

- Check for ewe debility, illness.
- Check for weak lambs resulting from abortion agents.

Localized oedema, no kidney autolysis, no thrombus, pointed end to artery indicate death late in parturition, i.e. dystocia.

- Check degree of supervision.
- Check shepherd knowledge and skill.
- Check breed of ewe and ram – disproportion.

Note: Meconium staining of coat may indicate fetal distress during parturition, or prolonged labour.

Postpartum deaths

Lungs uninflated or poorly inflated, thrombus at end of umbilical artery indicate immediate postpartum death.

- Check for injury during birth – fractured ribs, liver haemorrhage, brain haemorrhage.
- Check for prolonged parturition – anoxia, placental separation.
- Check for supervision at birth – asphyxia in membranes.
- Check for severe congenital abnormality.

Lungs inflated, foot membranes still present indicate lamb has breathed but not walked:

- Check for dystocia causing brain damage – especially large single. These rapidly succumb to hypothermia because they are unable to control body temperature.
- Check for severe swayback – cavitation of brain may be visible macroscopically.
- Check for border disease – fleece changes, tremors in live lamb.
- Check for other congenital abnormality, e.g. cerebellar hypoplasia – abnormally high head carriage or opisthotonus in live lamb.
- Check for severe nutritional myopathy – white streaks in muscles, blood sample ewes for glutathione peroxidase (GSH-Px).

Lamb has walked (foot membranes absent), empty gastrointestinal tract, meconium may not be expelled, brown fat partially or completely metabolized indicate failure to feed.

- Check degree of postpartum supervision.
- Check for one of multiples especially triplets.
- Check ewe udder – mastitis.
- Check for mismothering, rejection, inexperienced mother.
- Check for extreme chilling – lack of shelter, severe weather.
- Check for congenital abnormality – e.g. cleft palate.

Lambs dying at more than 1 day of age (fetal fluids dried, navel partly or completely dry).

The most important cause is hypothermia (exposure and/or starvation). The now common use of a stomach tube for feeding may give a false impression of the lamb not having starved. Recent feeding by stomach tube may be indicated by presence of liquid milk rather than clot, no absorption into lacteals, and metabolism of brown fat reserves.

- Check for starvation – empty gastrointestinal tract (unless stomach tubed as above), brown fat stores metabolized. This is most likely to arise from lack of colostrum due to mismothering, undernutrition of ewe, large litter, udder abnormality.
- Check for exposure – in addition to empty gastrointestinal tract and brown fat metabolism, there is usually some yellow-coloured oedema of the extremities. Bad weather and lack of shelter are the common causes.
- Check for subclinical copper deficiency – lambs may be of low viability, succumbing to hypothermia, and yet not show swayback.

Note: The amount of colostrum required to prevent hypothermia is estimated to be 180–210 ml/kg body weight in 24 h, depending on weather conditions, housing, etc. If insufficient ewe colostrum is available, goat or cow colostrum may be substituted. Care should be taken that colostrum from only CAE tested goats is used for maedi-accredited flocks. If cow colostrum is used, the possibility of anaemia developing in some lambs should be noted. See chapter 17.

If muzzle is wet, abomasum filled with saliva and gas, and often meconium not expelled, indicate watery mouth.

- Check for supervision of colostrum intake – amount and delay after birth.

This condition is now thought to be a result of the action of bacterial endotoxins produced in lambs with a delayed or inadequate colostrum intake. Research indicates that lambs which have received colostrum within 30 min of birth do not succumb to watery mouth. It is probable that 150–200 ml of good quality colostrum, i.e. from the first milking, are adequate to prevent this condition (but *not* enough to prevent hypothermia – see above).

If enteritis or dehydration is present:

- Check for digestive scour.
- Check for *E. coli* scour.
- Check for lamb dysentery.
- Check for *Salmonella*.
- Check for *Rotavirus*.
- Check for cryptosporidia.

Laboratory tests are likely to be required for confirmation of diagnosis. For full details, see chapter 10.

If signs of local or generalized infection (neonatal septicaemia) are present, e.g. navel infection, joint infection, liver abscess, spinal abscess.

- Check for hygiene at lambing.
- Check lambing pens – cleaning out, bedding, etc.
- Check for technique of routine navel disinfection (a quick squirt with a purple spray may not be adequate in the face of pathogenic bacteria, or iodine dip may be poured back into stock bottle after use).
- Check colostrum intake – volume and timing. Check serum samples from several lambs for IgG content. Values <20 mg/ml indicate inadequate colostrum supply or delayed intake, <30 mg/ml indicate moderate supply, <40 mg/ml good supply. Zinc sulphate turbidity test is an alternative – <20 units indicates poor or delayed uptake.
- Check for possible subclinical copper deficiency – such lambs may be of low viability, yet not showing swayback, and may succumb more easily to infections.
- In tick area, check for tick pyaemia.

Laboratory tests are likely to be required if the pathogen is to be identified. Whilst common organisms such as *E. coli*, *Staph. aureus* and *F. necrophorum* are likely to be found in many cases, other organisms such as *Listeria*, *Chlamydia*, mycoplasmas, *Erysipelothrix* and streptococci may be responsible, and their isolation will affect treatment.

Other common causes of neonatal deaths

(1) Predation – care should be taken to distinguish whether this occurred before death and was a contributing factor, or whether it occurred after death. If before death, there should be signs of bruising and haemorrhage at the damaged sites.

Note that lambs weak for other reasons are most likely to succumb to predators, e.g. foxes, or crows which peck out eyes.

(2) Inhalation pneumonia – this may occur where weak lambs are fed with a bottle, where a stomach tube is used incorrectly, i.e. placed in the trachea or too high up the oesophagus, or where a moribund lamb is fed by stomach tube and regurgitation takes place (such lambs have no swallowing reflex).

(3) Severe gingival orf – starvation is the usual cause of death in such cases.

(4) Nutritional myopathy (selenium/vitamin E deficiency). In some affected flocks, lambs may be weak or unable to stand at birth. White streaks or patches should be visible in skeletal or cardiac muscle, and diagnosis can be confirmed by histology and GSH-Px estimations in same group.

(5) Anaemia caused by feeding cow colostrum – this condition should be suspected if the carcase is pale with very watery blood. Deaths occur at 1–3 weeks of age. See chapter 17.

(6) Trauma – this is a common cause of death, particularly fractured ribs caused by treading by ewes if housed.

(7) Overlying – again in housed animals. Lambs are simply found dead, but if careful attention is paid to the head, this often appears flattened where it was trapped by the ewe sitting on it.

9 Inadequate growth rate

Estimation of optimum growth rates
Inadequate birth weights
Poor early growth
Poor growth in transitional milk to grass
    period
Late lactation period
Post-weaning growth retardation (ill thrift)
    Nutritional
    Parasitism
    Chronic disease
Poor growth on complete diets

This field is one which most commonly gives rise to complaint by sheep keepers and yet is the most difficult in which to give a quick and easy solution. Rarely, if ever, is the cause simple or indeed single. Nothing other than optimum growth rates will satisfy the owner, but by the time it is apparent that the flock is falling short of this aim, pathological change, if present, may have progressed to a point which will require time to correct. The end result may be conflict and dissatisfaction to all, including the bank manager!

But what is the optimum growth rate? The clinician *must* be able to arrive at an independent decision as to the presence or absence of depressed growth rates. To do this, one must be very familiar with normal growth rates for breed, age, management system, season, and nutritional inputs as well as the probable effects on growth of any disease which may be involved.

Estimation of optimum growth rate

The following factors will be relevant.

Birth weights

- Are these adequate for the breed or cross? (Can be estimated as the mean for the parent breeds plus any heterosis effect.)
- Presence of disease affecting birth weight and early growth, e.g. copper deficiency, border disease, other forms of abortion.
- Placental competition in prolific ewes.

Food conversion rates

- 1:1 may be achieved during early milk nutrition.
- With the change to grass-based nutrition, it then falls rapidly and may be as low as 10:1 on very poor quality forages.
- The newer 'complete' feeds for lamb finishing may be as good as 3:1.

Target weights

- Prime finished lamb – 18 kg carcase at 20 weeks. (Estimated dead carcase weight is usually 1–2 kg less than half live weight, but early fast growing lambs can kill out at 50% or even higher.) With a birth weight of 4–5 kg this requires a growth rate of a minimum of 1.5 kg per week. Fast growing single lambs can achieve double this.

- Breed replacements should achieve 60% of mature weight at 36 weeks if they are to be mated as ewe lambs. If the mature weight is 75 kg, this requires an average weight gain of 1.4 kg per week.

Projected grass output

If the client is able to offer the necessary information, it may be possible to assess output against a true target as follows:

Total liveweight gain per hectare = (total forage output × DM × utilization × digestibility × conversion rate × stocking rate).

Growth rate is a function of the availability, absorption and utilization of inputs over and above those required for basal metabolic rate under prevailing environmental conditions. It follows that suboptimal growth rates are a result of the following:

- inadequate inputs (quantity and/or quality),
- reduced appetite (parasites),
- accelerated throughput (scouring),
- protein loss into intestine or urine,
- excessive demands (raised basal metabolic rate in adverse weather conditions).

Frequently there will be a combination of several of these factors.

It is this potentially complex equation which makes the diagnosis and treatment of the causes of inadequate growth rate or ill thrift so difficult.

In the development of the growing lamb, there are two distinct divisions of the nature of food inputs, and therefore two phases of potential reductions in growth rate. These are the 'milk dominated', and 'grass dominated' phases. In addition, modern husbandry methods include complete feeding of housed lambs. Figure 9.1 lists the causes of inadequate growth rates in lambs and the tests possible.

Milk dominated feed period

Inadequate birth weights

This subject is discussed under suboptimal reproductive performance (chapter 2) and perinatal mortality (chapter 8), but is also of significance in this present area of consideration.

76

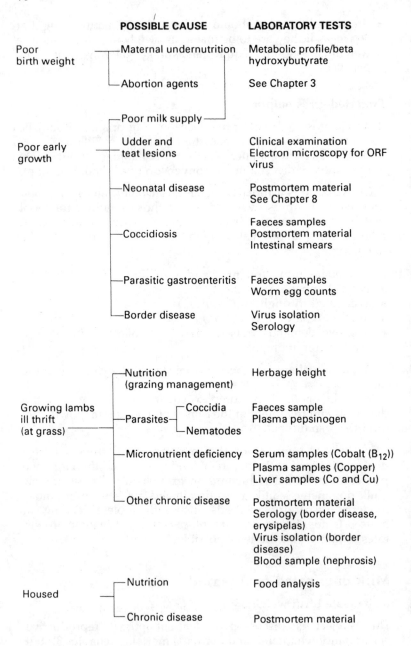

POSSIBLE CAUSE	LABORATORY TESTS

Poor birth weight
— Maternal undernutrition — Metabolic profile/beta hydroxybutyrate
— Abortion agents — See Chapter 3

— Poor milk supply —

Poor early growth
Udder and teat lesions — Clinical examination / Electron microscopy for ORF virus

— Neonatal disease — Postmortem material / See Chapter 8

— Coccidiosis — Faeces samples / Postmortem material / Intestinal smears

— Parasitic gastroenteritis — Faeces samples / Worm egg counts

— Border disease — Virus isolation / Serology

Growing lambs ill thrift (at grass)
— Nutrition (grazing management) — Herbage height

— Parasites — Coccidia / Nematodes — Faeces sample / Plasma pepsinogen

— Micronutrient deficiency — Serum samples (Cobalt (B$_{12}$)) / Plasma samples (Copper) / Liver samples (Co and Cu)

— Other chronic disease — Postmortem material / Serology (border disease, erysipelas) / Virus isolation (border disease) / Blood sample (nephrosis)

Housed
— Nutrition — Food analysis

— Chronic disease — Postmortem material

Figure 9.1 Inadequate growth rates

Low birth weight lambs may arise as a result of
- prematurity due to non-infective conditions,
- prematurity as a result of infectious agents such as *Toxoplasma*, *Chlamydia*, etc. causing subcritical placentitis,
- restricted placental development in large litters,
- early fetal loss.

Whatever the cause, low birth weight lambs often have a poor sucking drive, or are unable to compete with stronger lambs for available milk. They are thus disadvantaged both from total milk intake, and often reduced immunoglobulin intake. It is a common observation that these lambs take a noticeably longer time to reach adequate weights than normal contemporaries.

Individual or sporadic low birth weight lambs

- Check possibility of early fetal loss. This results in poor placentation for the surviving embryos, since the caruncles which would have been utilized by the dead embryos do not become available to the survivors. This is commonly the explanation for the birth of lambs of widely differing birth weights to the same ewe. Examination of the placenta may show few cotyledons (the normal number is about 40 per horn) or abnormally small cotyledons.
- Check health and condition of ewe – underfeeding or debility give poor lamb weights.

Many low birth weight lambs

- Check if is highly prolific flock – limited placentation available for each fetus.
- Check for inadequate ewe nutrition in early pregnancy causing poor placentation (difficult to establish at this stage, but size of cotyledons may give guide).
- Check for inadequate ewe nutrition in late pregnancy – overestimate of winter grass quality, failure to feed concentrates, poor concentrates.
- Check for abortion agent operating in flock. See chapter 3.

Inadequate growth during milk dominated nutrition

At this stage, poor growth is usually a reflection of inadequate milk supply, although the presence of neonatal disease within the flock will obviously also have an effect.

Individual lambs showing poor growth

- Check milk supply – mastitis, teat lesions, competition if one of multiple.
- Check for mismothering or rejection (may follow rounding up for dosing, etc.).
- Check ability to suck – mouth lesions (severe orf affecting the gums may not be noticed unless inside of mouth is examined).
- Check for disease – neonatal septicaemia, joint ill.
- Check for nephrosis – blood sample for urea and creatinine estimation. Lambs are dull, anorexic and afebrile with increased thirst for water. The cause is not known. PME usually shows enlarged pale kidneys, although histology may be required to confirm some cases.
- Check for possibility of 'wool or milk ball' in abomasum – may be detectable on palpation.

Note: Poor growth plus green 'grass' type liquid faeces in the first 4 weeks of life indicate an inadequate milk supply. It may be difficult for the client to accept this.

Many lambs showing poor growth rates

During the early part of the 'milk' nutrition phase, this is almost invariably due to poor milk supply, following inadequate nutrition of the ewe flock both during late pregnancy and early lactation. If optimal peak lactation is not reached very soon after parturition, it will never be attained. Since optimum growth rate is initiated at this critical time (with very high conversion rates if the supply is adequate), this must be the first area of investigation. Often client resistance will be evident, since there is inevitably some reflection on management. The other common cause of poor performance in the 2–8 week stage is coccidiosis. Although scouring would normally be expected to be a major feature of heavy infections, some lambs may simply show ill thrift with poor open wool.

   Where a significant number of lambs are affected, it is always worth sacrificing a small number of typical cases to assist in reaching an accurate diagnosis.

- Check ewe condition and nutrition – before and after lambing.
- Check litter size of affected lambs. If prolific flock, may be poor management of triplets.
- Check for prolonged wet or cold weather with high chill factor.

- Check for coccidiosis – oocyst count is not reliable (see chapter 10).
- Check for copper deficiency. Subclinical deficiency may exist without evidence of 'swayback' lambs. May lead to poor viability of lambs, with poor sucking instincts and higher susceptibility to disease. Take blood samples (minimum six animals) and liver samples for copper estimation.
- Check for border disease – characteristic hairy shakers are diagnostic, but may not always be present. Blood samples for virus isolation.
- Check for orf infection of lambs' lips and ewes' teats.
- Check for evidence of other disease restricting mobility, or after effects of neonatal disease.
- Check for nephrosis as above.

Transitional milk to grass period

Frequently this period (from 4–5 weeks of age) will coincide with imposed limitations of forage supply, much of the available area being closed for forage conservation. Several factors follow from this.

The owner may underestimate the demand by the lamb crop for grass, planning stocking rates for adults only. By the time it is apparent that forage is short, the stock are several days overdue for a move. This both delays the onset of full grazing by the lamb crop, and produces a degree of malnutrition, hence reduced growth.

The same limitation of grazing will require the lambs to take in grass contaminated with both coccidial oocysts and, unless clean grazing is available, infective nematode larvae. These last two factors are considered in chapter 10 as important causes of scouring, but also have major effects on growth rates.

Even where adequate grass appears to be available, large mobs of sheep may cause poaching or spoilage, particularly in wet weather, drastically reducing palatability and utilization.

- Check for stocking rate and grass length (4–6 cm is optimal)
- Where set stocking is used, grass availability must be carefully monitored, with buffer areas available for grazing or conservation according to growing conditions.
- Check for provision of creep feed if grazing is inadequate.
- Check for parasitic disease – faeces samples for oocysts and nematode eggs (chapter 10).

Note: Where mixed infections of coccidiosis and *Nematodirus* occur, losses can be significant with a major effect on growth rate of survivors.

Grass nutrition period to weaning

In contrast to milk, which is a more or less standard product as far as nutrient content is concerned, the nutrient value of grazing varies widely. This ranges from the short dense rapidly growing specific 'sheep' mixture of the intensive lowland unit, to the low nutrient value of the high hill. It is important that the practitioner recognizes this variability in quality as well as quantity, and the effect on both intake and growth rates. The effects of parasitism, particularly parasitic gastroenteritis and nematodiriasis, are again major factors if clean or safe grazing is not available. In addition the effects of any micronutrient deficiency begin to be seen, although they assume a greater significance after weaning.

- Check quality and quantity of forage before searching for more exotic causes.
- Check for low dry matter content. This may directly limit nutrient availability for optimum growth.
- If no clean or safe pastures have been available for the ewe and lamb post lambing, check faeces samples for coccidia and nematode egg count. See remarks above re mixed coccidiosis and *Nematodirus* infection. The usual upper age limits for these infections are about 8 weeks for coccidiosis and 12 weeks for *Nematodirus*.

Post-weaning growth retardation (ill thrift)

Although the occasional individual case will occur due to chronic infection contracted at an earlier stage, the vast majority of incidents will affect significant numbers of lambs within a group or flock. These cases pose perhaps some of the most difficult diagnostic problems in sheep clinical work, since the causes are almost invariably multifactorial. This is often combined with client resistance to the more obvious solutions. The cry 'But I have been worming them every three weeks' often echoes through the sheep clinician's dreams!

The only solution for a successful diagnosis is that the clinician works methodically through the possibilities.

The main causes of poor performance at this stage of the production cycle are:

- nutritional,
- acute gastrointestinal parasite damage,
- chronic after effects of parasitism,
- micronutrient deficiency,
- chronic disease, e.g. erysipelas, border disease, pasteurellosis.

Some of these will be accompanied by other symptoms which help to narrow the field, e.g. scouring (see chapter 10), lameness (chapter 14).

Check for nutritional causes

There may be an inadequate supply of forage if the season has been difficult for conservation. Check the amount and type of pasture available and grazing history since weaning. In late autumn this age group of lambs is often grazed on cattle pasture, which may be of poor palatibility. The value of autumn and winter grazing is often overestimated. Check also for slurry or manure spreading which greatly reduces palatability.

Note: Pasture spread with pig slurry is dangerous because of the high copper content, and may induce copper poisoning.

Check for parasitic causes

In this age group, chronic gastrointestinal parasitism is the most common cause of failure to thrive. Although anthelmintics may be administered regularly, reinfection occurs immediately if contaminated pasture is being grazed, and repeated damage is caused by the developing larvae. *Negative results for nematode eggs in faeces samples from such animals do not exclude the possibility of chronic worm damage.*

If samples are negative, check for recent worming (prepatent period is about 3 weeks, so animals wormed within that time will show negative counts).

Blood samples for pepsinogen and albumin content may also assist in indicating chronic gastric damage.

Note: Poor growth, linked to chronic parasitism, has been shown to be due to depression of appetite, with reduced food intake as well as increased nitrogen loss into intestine and urine.

If poor growth rates are experienced with clean or safe grazing systems, check past grazing history for evidence of inadvertent contamination.

Note: Mixed graxing or alternate grazing with cattle and sheep is now known to allow the possibility of breakdowns, especially with *Nematodirus*, as calves are able to act as hosts.

Check for micronutrient deficiencies

Deficiencies of cobalt (pine) and copper are both implicated as causes of ill thrift in this age group. Local knowledge of geology and disease patterns should assist the clinician in deciding the possible involvement of these trace elements, but even so the diagnosis is by no means straightforward.

Apparently healthy, thriving animals may be found to have marginal or low blood values, and unthrifty animals may have apparently normal values. In the end, the clinician may have to rely on response to treatment as the final diagnostic feature (if the temptation to treat with everything 'in case' is resisted).

Cobalt
Cobalt deficiency produces poor growth, weakness and emaciation. Lambs are anaemic, become anorexic and often show a watery discharge from the eyes. Cobalt is an essential component of vitamin B_{12}, which is manufactured by the rumen microflora.

● Check serum vitamin B_{12} (clotted blood sample) <0.15 pmol/ ml indicates deficiency.
● Check liver B_{12} if samples available <0.09 μmol/kg wet weight indicates deficiency.
● Check urine sample for formiminoglutamic acid (FIGLU) and methylmalonic acid (MMA) – these are abnormal metabolites of propionic acid which accumulate in Co deficiency.
● Check herbage and soil cobalt content – <1.9 μmol/kg in diet and <5 μmol/kg soil indicate deficiency.
● Test dose a group of affected animals and monitor weight gain against untreated group.

Copper
Copper deficiency produces effects on the wool (loss of crimp – steely wool), depressed growth and anaemia. It is usually only seen where hill grazing has been improved by draining and liming. In this situation, the copper deficiency is induced by increased availability of minerals in the pasture – molybdenum, iron and sulphur, which are ingested in soil taken in with the herbage.

- Check plasma copper concentration (heparinized sample): <9.5 μmol/l indicates deficiency, but is less accurate than liver concentration.
- Check liver copper concentration – this gives a better indication of true copper status than plasma – <160 μmol/kg DM indicates deficiency.
- Check blood sample for superoxide dismutase (SOD) concentration – low value indicates prolonged deficiency (normal value in lambs is 0.4–0.5 i.u./mg Hb).
- Check herbage and soil analyses for copper, molybdenum and sulphur content, although these can be difficult to interpret if pasture improvement (which increases Mo and S availability and decreases Cu availability) has taken place. Specialist help may be required in interpretation.

Selenium
Selenium deficiency causes ill thrift in lambs in New Zealand and Australia, but has not yet been implicated in the UK.

Other chronic diseases

- Check for border disease (blood sample for virus isolation). This may affect flocks without the appearance of characteristic hairy shaker lambs. Affected lambs are stunted and often show diarrhoea.
- Check for nephrosis – as previously stated, the cause is not established. In some cases it may be associated with *Nematodirus* infection, and dehydration after severe scouring, but this is not always the case (blood sample for urea and creatinine concentrations).
- Check for chronic erysipelas (serology).
- Check for chronic pasteurellosis.
- If lambs are retained late in the season, check for subclinical liver fluke.

Finishing lambs on 'complete' diets

This now common method of finishing lambs is highly cost effective and, under good management, gives the opportunity to monitor accurately growth and food conversion rates. Suboptimal growth rates should therefore be apparent at a much earlier stage than under less carefully controlled grass based systems.

- Check analysis of diet and cost. Low cost almost certainly means poor quality.
- Check fibre and ash content – high values mean poorer quality (note though, that diets including processed straw will be higher in fibre but still acceptable). If in doubt check with manufacturer for ingredients and expected growth rates.
- Check feeding routine – freshness of supply. Soiled or stale food will not be eaten.
- Check for change in batch – different palatability.
- Check for trough space allowed.
- Check for uniformity of age groups, size of animals.
- Check house for ventilation – heat stress or excessive humidity.
- Check for bedding quantity and dryness – possible ammonia build-up.
- Check water supply – sheep are particularly susceptible to rejection of water supply if soiled.
- Check for too rapid introduction of feed, chronic acidosis.
- Check for concurrent disease especially atypical pneumonia.

All losses should be checked by postmortem examination for signs of chronic lung disease, or other feed-associated problems such as urolithiasis.

10 Diarrhoea

Neonatal diarrhoea
  Dietary
  Infections
Diarrhoea in growing lambs
  Dietary
  Parasitism
  Infections
  Toxins
Breakdown of clean or safe grazing systems
Diarrhoea in store lambs
Diarrhoea in adults
  Without weight loss
  With weight loss
  With systemic disease

Normal faeces in the sheep can vary from hard pellets to a paste-like consistency, mainly as a result of variations in the water content of the diet, but there is also some individual and breed variation. Liquid faeces are a reflection of increased fluid passage from the lower intestine, and not in themselves proof of the existence of pathological change or overt disease. Since the sheep requires some 2.5% of body weight in dry matter intake daily for maintenance, the demand for nutrients may lead

Table 10.1 Scouring – common causes

Age group	Type	Cause	Clinical features
Neonatal	Digestive		Generally not ill
	Infective	E. coli	
		Salmonella	Generally ill, dehydration rapid
		Rotavirus	
		Cryptosporidia	
		Clostridia	Severe illness or sudden death
Growing lambs	Dietary	Milk supply failure	Premature 'grass' faeces. Failure to thrive
		Low dry matter grass	Persistent scour
		High nitrogen in grass	Less effect on growth rate
		Overeating	Characteristic faeces, ill, rumen stasis
	Infective	Salmonella	Ill. Associated with abortions in ewes
		Border disease	Not ill, but ill thrift, persistent scour
	Parasitic	Coccidiosis	Severe scour. Haemorrhagic. Deaths. Ill thrift
		Nematodirus	in survivors
		Parasitic gastroenteritis	Ill thrift. Deaths if neglected
	Toxic	Nitrates	Methaemoglobinaemia
Adults	Dietary	Overeating	Characteristic faeces, ill, rumen stasis
		Low dry matter intake	Not ill. Little effect on body weight
		Forage spoilage	Reluctance to eat
	Parasitic	Ostertagia II	Young ewes or rams.
		Trichostrongylus	Loss of weight Anaemia
	Infective	Salmonella	Ill. Abortions in flock.
		Johnes	Sporadic, weight loss

Table 10.2 Scouring – aids to diagnosis

	Gross pathology	Microbiology	Parasitology	Haematology/ biochemistry
Neonatal enteritis	Enteritis/ septicaemia	E. coli Salmonella Clostridia Rotavirus	Cryptosporidia oocysts	IgG status - Zn turbidity
Coccidiosis	Lower small intestine Colon – dysentery	–	Faecal oocysts Intestinal smear Species differen- tiation	Packed cell volume
Parasitic gastro- enteritis	Abomasum – Ostertagia Haemonchus. Trichostrongylus Small intestine – Trichostrongylus Nematodirus (dysentery)	–	Egg counts Worm counts Mucosal ·scrape	Plasma pepsinogen. Packed cell volume
Nitrate poisoning	Brown blood	–	–	Methaemoglo- binaemia
Acidosis	Rumen contents/pH	–	–	–
Johnes	Thickened lower small intestine. Yellow pigment sometimes	Smear Histology Repeated faeces sampling	–	AGID/ Complement fixation test

to total fluid intake beyond the capacity of the gastrointestinal tract to reabsorb fluid when on a low dry matter diet. Diarrhoea is, therefore the end result of either increased fluid intake (either because of increased thirst, or low dry matter intake) or of reduced reabsorption, and/or fluid loss into the intestine.

Increased thirst may result from normal physiological proces-ses such as pregnancy or lactation. It also results from the attempt to maintain tissue fluid normality after electrolyte loss, or may follow increased electrolyte intake, e.g. in feed blocks. Low dry matter intake is very common, especially in the autumn grass flush, but can also result from feeding poor quality wet silage or excessive amounts of roots.

A combination of reduced reabsorption from the lumen of the intestine, and increased fluid loss through damaged mucosa into the intestine is found in many forms of both gastroenteritis and inflammatory change in the lower intestine, ranging from bacterial infections such as *E. coli* and *Salmonella*, to parasitic diseases such as coccidiosis and parasitic gastroenteritis.

Scouring itself does not comprise a threat to life, except in the newborn, if fluid loss and electrolyte loss are compensated for by increased intake, and provided that there is no major damage to intestinal mucosa. It is necessarily much more serious in the neonate, with its poor thermoregulatory abilities and lack of large fluid reserves in tissues and rumen. The adult, on the other hand, having the advantage in all these factors, can and does compensate, frequently suffering only marginal reductions in production.

The many causes of scouring are commonly both age and diet related (see Table 10.1), thus in the investigation of any particular incident, many conditions can be excluded on these grounds alone. Aids to the diagnosis of scouring are given in Table 10.2.

Lambs from birth to 4 weeks

Scouring in the neonate can be subdivided into infectious and digestive causes for the purpose of diagnosis. The two groups may be distinguished by the severity of the general symptoms shown, rather than the type or appearance of the faeces. In addition, digestive scour may affect individual animals or a small group, whereas an infectious agent will usually affect many or all lambs. Infectious forms are more commonly encountered towards the end of the lambing period, particularly in housed flocks, as a result of a build-up of infection.

The following organisms are those most commonly responsible for enteritis in the neonatal lamb:

Bacteria

E. coli

Salmonella spp.

Cl. perfringens type B

Campylobacter

Viruses

Rotavirus

The significance of other viruses in the UK is not known. Enteroviruses, reoviruses, adenoviruses and astrovirus have been isolated from lamb faeces.

Protozoon

Cryptosporidium

Differentiation of the specific causal agent in any individual outbreak will usually be difficult on clinical grounds alone. Although the field can be narrowed to some degree, the clinician must at all times be prepared to obtain laboratory confirmation of the presence of any specific factor. Some outbreaks will involve significant lamb mortality, and full use should be made of any available postmortem material. See chapter 8 for further details.

The following points will be a guide to the possible cause of any particular incident, in association with laboratory findings. The possibility of mixed infections should also be borne in mind, and if laboratory tests or response to therapy indicate a complex aetiology, appropriate action should be taken.

Lambs not ill, appetite maintained, dehydration not severe

● Check for digestive scour.

Digestive scour, which often has a pasty white appearance, is usually associated with artificial feeding or supplementation of lambs of ewes with an inadequate milk supply. Lambs do not exhibit the rapid and severe depression which usually accompanies infectious forms of scour, and provided the lamb continues to suck, the end result may not be serious.

● Check for excess milk intake, e.g. loss of a twin.
● Check management of artificially reared lambs – type of milk substitute, correct mixing, feeding temperature, amount per feed, frequency of feeding.
● Check hygiene and cleaning of feeders.

Note: Lambs can be reared very satisfactorily on *ad libitum* cold feeding systems. There is often the temptation to top up with warm milk, but this should be resisted, as it leads to fluctuations in the temperature of the milk which may cause digestive problems. Female lambs on *ad libitum* feeding occasionally exhibit urine scalding, which superficially may give the appearance of scouring.

Lambs show profuse bloody scour, abdominal pain and rapid death

● Check for lamb dysentery.
● Check vaccination history.

Often affects the strongest lambs. Postmortem picture is pathognomonic – severe enteritis affecting ileum; necrotic mucosa, serous or bloodstained fluid in peritoneum. For confirmation submit intestinal contents (30 ml) to laboratory for direct smear, or ELISA (enzyme-linked immunosorbent assay).

Lambs show severe scour (often greenish colour), septicaemia and death; illness and abortions in ewes

- Check for salmonellosis – bacteriological examination of faeces, rectal swabs and carcases (posterior mesenteric lymph nodes are particularly useful).

Lambs show profuse scour, weakness and dehydration

It is this group which gives the most difficulty in diagnosis. The lambs are very susceptible to dehydration, and a specific diagnosis is essential for the selection of appropriate treatment, and yet laboratory diagnosis must inevitably take some time. The nature of the faeces and the severity of the depression are of little assistance.

- Check for enterotoxigenic *E. coli* (ETEC) – indirect fluorescence antibody test (IFAT) on fresh sample of small intestine, culture, bacterial counts ($> 10^8/g$ of intestinal contents), identification of K99 antigen.

Note: Although cases of watery mouth may occur in a flock affected by ETEC, scouring is not a common feature of this condition.

- Check for salmonellosis as above.
- Check for *Rotavirus* – faeces sample for electron microscopy, ELISA, IFAT.
- Check for *Campylobacter* – not usually thought to be a significant problem in lambs.

Lambs ill from 4 days approximately, afebrile, anorectic

- Check for *Cryptosporidium* – faecal smears stained with Giemsa for detection of oocysts (these are much smaller than coccidial oocysts), histology of small and large intestines.

Note: Although *Cryptosporidium* is a protozoon, the short life cycle (2–4 days) gives the appearance of a bacterial infection.

The parasite is not host specific, therefore it can be contracted from calves for example. It is also a zoonosis.

Growing lambs

With increasing age, the lamb is less susceptible to the acute dehydration of scouring, except in the case of severe damage such as that produced by acute nematodiriasis. When the full transfer to grass-based nutrition takes place, the fluid reserves of the rumen and large intestine become available to buffer the effects of scouring. However, in addition to the chronic intestinal damage persisting after neonatal infections, the lamb frequently has to adapt to very low dry matter forage intake, as well as the challenge of parasitic diseases such as coccidiosis and helminthiasis.

In addition, chronic intestinal damage with erosion of villi leads to long-term malabsorption, protein leakage and chronic anaemia, giving severe diagnostic problems over the long term. Conflict with the client concerning aetiology and perceived failure to respond to treatment is common.

The following causes of scouring in growing lambs should be considered:

Dietary
  Milk supply failure
  Premature dependence on grass
  Nitrogenous or other fertilizer ingestion
  Overfeeding/acidosis
Bacterial
  Salmonella
  Campylobacter
Virus Border disease
Parasites
  Coccidiosis
  Nematodirus
  Parasitic gastroenteritis
Toxins
  Molybdenum ⎤
  Copper | Worth considering only in special
  Lead | circumstances, or if more common
  Ragwort ⎦ causes eliminated.

At this stage, the incidence, i.e. individuals or whole groups affected, and any history of prolonged housing or heavy stocking on lambing paddocks will be of significance.

Individuals or small numbers affected

- Check ewe for milk supply failure – teat lesions or mastitis. Such lambs have severely reduced growth rates, a 'potbellied' appearance, and have a 'grass scour' before the age at which they should be totally grass dependent.
- Check for fibre-filled abomasum (palpate) as result of above.
- If artificially reared, check for weaning too early before rumen adequately developed.

Many lambs or whole groups affected

Although dietary factors may be implicated, parasitic disease is the most common cause.

- Check for coccidiosis.

The diagnosis of coccidiosis is not a straightforward matter. Perfectly healthy lambs may show very high faecal oocyst counts (1×10^6/g), whilst severe pathological lesions may be present in lambs showing negligible or low counts. This anomaly can be explained by two factors.

(1) The infection may be with relatively non-pathogenic species of coccidia, e.g. *Eimeria bakuensis*. These infect the cells of the small intestine causing little damage to the crypt stem cells, and minor amounts of damage can be compensated for within the large intestine.
(2) Pathogenic species, *E. crandallis* and particularly *E. ovinoidalis*, which infect the lower small intestine, caecum and colon may cause severe damage to crypt cells early in the life cycle, before there is any significant production of oocysts. In addition the period of maximum oocyst production is short, so that samples taken late in an infection may also show low counts.

Confirmation of diagnosis rests upon demonstration of a combination of the following factors:

- age of affected lambs 4–7 weeks,
- lambs housed for extended period after birth, or
- lambs and ewes kept tightly stocked after lambing,
- severe diarrhoea often with blood,
- some lambs show tenesmus,
- some lambs with oocyst counts $>1 \times 10^5$/g,

- species present are *E. crandallis* and/or *E. ovinoidalis* (differentiation of oocysts is a specialist laboratory task),
- postmortem examination shows lesions in lower small intestine, caecum and colon – raised white spots, mucosa thickened and inflamed,
- smears of intestinal scrapings show presence of developing stages of coccidia.

Note: Response to treatment with sulphonamides is not diagnostic, since these have a wide range of action against other infectious agents.

- Check for *Nematodirus battus* infection.

This is caused by sudden mass hatching of infective larvae on pasture contaminated by young lambs grazing the pasture the previous year. Hatching follows a rise in temperature to above 10°C following a period of cold sensitization. Forecasts of disease are based on weather conditions together with timing. Disease will occur if the mass hatching coincides with the presence of susceptible lambs on the pasture. If hatching occurs early in the season before the lambs are eating significant quantities of grass, or if hatching is very late when lambs are past the most susceptible age, disease is not likely. Disease due to *N. battus* is rare in lambs over 3 months of age, but *N. filicollis* can cause disease in hogs in autumn.

Diagnosis is based on the following:

- sudden onset of severe scouring,
- grazing history – land grazed by lambs in previous year,
- seasonal forecast of disease,
- lambs are dull, dehydrated, sometimes show abdominal pain,
- faeces sample may show characteristic *Nematodirus* eggs, but lambs may be ill before many are present, as developing immature worms do severe damage,
- some deaths will occur,
- PME shows acute enteritis with worms present in the intestine (look like cottonwool on mucosa).

Note: Concurrent infection with coccidiosis may increase the pathogenicity of *Nematodirus*.
Note: Although nematodiriasis is classically a spring problem, outbreaks of scouring and weight loss caused by *N. filicollis* are sometimes seen in autumn.

- Check for parasitic gastroenteritis.

This is still the major source of loss in growing lambs. The main species of helminths involved are *Ostertagia* spp. and *Trichostrongylus* spp.

Note: *Haemonchus* infection usually causes severe anaemia, oedema and weakness. It is not usually associated with scouring.

Cooperia, *Strongyloides* and *Bunostomum* may be found in the small intestine but rarely in sufficient numbers to be pathogenic.

Parasites of the large intestine (*Oesophagostomum*, *Chabertia* and *Trichuris*) are rarely present in sufficient numbers to be pathogenic.

Note: All the above worm species cannot be distinguished in a routine worm egg count, since the eggs are virtually indistinguishable (although computer-aided identification may be a technique available in the future). Differentiation requires larval culture, or examination of eggs by a very experienced parasitologist.

Diagnosis is based on the following criteria:

- scouring and weight loss from July onwards,
- grazing history – contaminated pasture,
- anthelmintic treatment programme – inadequate or infrequent dosing early in the season when on contaminated grazing, allows a build-up of infective larvae by early summer,
- egg counts of undosed lambs (may be >1000 eggs per gram),
- raised plasma pepsinogen concentration (>1 i.u./litre),
- *Ostertagia* causes characteristic abomasal lesions (raised nodules in thickened mucosa),
- *Trichostrongylus* causes enteritis, hypertrophy of mucosa with flattened areas in long-standing cases,
- presence of large numbers of worms at PME – 10 000–15 000 *Ostertagia*, 20 000–30 000 *Trichostrongylus* (*Ostertagia* are easily visible in abomasum, but hair-like *Trichostrongylus* in small intestine can easily be overlooked.)

All the above conditions are involved in the ill thrift problem – see chapter 9.

Problems in diagnosis

Lambs may continue to scour after anthelmintic or anticoccidial treatment because of chronic damage to the intestine. The absence of parasites does not necessarily mean that they were not the original cause of the damage. Histological examination of the intestine usually shows erosion of villi, leading to malabsorption and protein leakage. It is often difficult to convince the client that parasitism has been involved when they say 'but I have wormed them regularly!' and faeces examinations are negative (often taken after a recent treatment with anthelmintic, anyway).

Resistance to anthelmintics may be blamed but, other than with *Haemonchus* infection, there is little evidence of resistance problems with modern anthelmintics in the UK as yet. Tests for resistance can be carried out if this is suspected. Faeces samples should be collected 7–10 days after worming with the correct dose of the anthelmintic under investigation. The presence of significant numbers of strongyle eggs indicates that further investigations should take place. Consult a laboratory for further assistance.

Breakdowns with 'clean' or 'safe' grazing systems

The introduction of safe grazing systems has been a major advance in parasite control where the farming system allows, but breakdowns frequently occur. Successful operation depends upon a clear knowledge of worm life cycles, effect of age, sex and pregnancy upon worm burdens, care with the timing and accuracy of drenching, and careful recording of grazing management.

- Check for transmission of *Nematodirus* via susceptible calves.
- Check for correct timing of anthelmintic treatments, i.e. immediately before turning on to clean pasture.
- Check for correct dosage with anthelmintic (gun calibration).
- Check area grazed by lambs in previous autumn.
- Check for transmission by unwormed groups, e.g. rams. These may carry a significant worm burden throughout the year unlike adult ewes.

Note: Although segments of the tapeworm *Monezia expansa* are commonly seen in the faeces of growing lambs, this parasite is thought not to have any pathogenic effects, other than very rarely causing physical obstruction of the intestine if present in large numbers.

If these parasitic conditions are eliminated as a cause of scouring the following conditions should be considered:

- Check for low dry matter forage intake, lush grass growth, excessive rainfall.

- Check for fertilizer application without rainfall.
- If housed, check for feed change, irregular water supply, excessive intake of concentrate feed (acidosis).
- Check for border disease – congenital infection can lead to poor thriving lambs showing chronic scour. See ill thrift in chapter 9.

Note: A nephrosis syndrome has recently been identified, with some affected lambs also showing black scour, rapid weight loss, fits, followed by death. Although the cause or causes are not yet known, one suggestion is a trickle-infection with *Nematodirus*.

Scouring in store lambs or young adults in late autumn/winter

Parasitic disease may again be a problem in this age group.

- Check for *Ostertagia* type II.
- Check for chronic *Trichostrongylus* infection.
- Check for *N. filicollis* infection.

Adult sheep

The same underlying factors apply to the control of the consistency of faecal material in the adult, as apply to younger animals, i.e. both physiological and pathological change will produce variation, which may or may not be of significance. In addition to the physiological variation of dry matter content of forage, the ewe will have the extra demands of pregnancy and lactation. Pregnancy will require extra nutrient intake to cope with the 'production' demand of fetal growth. If this is combined with forage of varying dry matter, especially silage, and of access to feed blocks with a high electrolyte (salt) content producing increased fluid intake, the result may well be continuously fluid faeces. Finally, the adult will be subject to greater risk of 'slow onset' conditions such as Johnes disease.

Sudden onset of scouring with systemic illness

- Check for salmonellosis.
- Check for concentrate overfeeding/acidosis.

Scouring with little significant weight loss

- Check for low dry matter intake – lush autumn grass, wet silage, roots, etc.
- Check for availability of thirst inducing mineral or feed blocks.
- Check for interrupted water supply or frozen water supply.
- This may be normal in some animals.

Scouring with weight loss

This may not be easily apparent if the starting point is from low body weight at the end of the lactation period.

Many cases or whole groups affected

- Check for *Trichostrongylus* infection.
- Check for *Ostertagia* type II.

Note: Haemonchosis usually causes rapid weight loss without scouring.

- Check for high N fertilizer application.

If fodder is available

- Check for conserved forage spoilage – mycotoxins.
- Check for other signs of listeriosis – scouring may precede onset of abortions or nervous signs.

If individuals or small numbers affected

- Check for Johnes disease – faeces samples, smear stained by Ziehl Neelson. (May need multiple samplings, and a negative result does not rule out the possibility of Johnes disease.) May require PME and smear of ileal mucosa or mesenteric lymph nodes, or histology of intestine to confirm diagnosis. The pigmented form is easily recognizable, with bright yellow coloration of the ileum.
- In autumn, check for access to acorns – excess intake causes black tarry scour followed by constipation.

Other occasional causes such as tumours will be diagnosed at PME only.

11 Tenesmus

Identification of system involved
    Alimentary
    Urinary
    Genital
Neonates
Growing lambs
Adult female
Adult male

This is a common sign in sheep (straining, striving, forcing), causing the sheep keeper to request assistance from the veterinarian. Unless the problem is obviously linked to parturition, the request is often in the form 'I have a sheep which is constipated'; this, almost invariably, is not the case! Thus, extra vigilance is needed, since to arrive at a considered diagnosis with which the owner will always disagree places the clinician in particular hazard.

The condition will usually be acute, and will have welfare implications as the animal will be suffering discomfort or pain. It will call for a rapid solution since, if not already present, continual tenesmus will often lead to prolapse of the rectum or vagina. On the other hand, except in outbreaks of urolithiasis or coccidiosis, cases will usually be limited to a single animal or small numbers, so the economic significance may be limited.

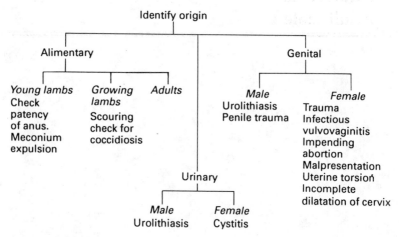

Figure 11.1 Tenesmus

The diagnostic procedure must always begin with the identification of the system involved (see Figure 11.1).

- Alimentary
- Urinary
- Genital

This will frequently not be obvious, except in the case of prolapse or a vaginal discharge. If the animal is a female of reproductive age and generally, but not inevitably, at some active stage of the reproductive cycle, the identification of the tract involved can usually be established by the use of a speculum. Alternatively, digital examination of, or insertion of a swab into, the vagina may be helpful. If no positive evidence emerges then a similar examination can be applied to the rectum.

As with much else in the diagnosis of disease in the sheep, the area for consideration can be narrowed by first establishing the sex and age group of the patient. This will eliminate many conditions.

Neonate

Note: Some lambs show tenesmus and cry with apparent pain when defaecating normally during the first few days of life.

- Check for failure to expel meconium. This is more commonly a cause of loss of appetite or a part of the 'watery mouth' syndrome.
- Check for tail adhesion due to dried meconium leading to a total seal of the anal ring.
- Check for congenital rectovaginal fistula. Usually only the vulva is patent.
- Check for imperforate anus. This usually causes abdominal distension rather than tenesmus.
- If castrated with rubber ring, check placement is not faulty.

Growing lamb (prepubertal)

Generally the cause of straining will be alimentary, and secondary to increased throughput of faecal material. This commonly results in irritation, inflammation and oedema of the rectal mucosa and anal sphincter, with persistent attempts to defaecate even with an empty rectum.

- Check for evidence of scouring, including faecal sample. Cause of scouring then to be investigated (Chapter 10).
- Check for coccidiosis. This is perhaps the most common cause, and will be one of the rare episodes when many animals will be affected.

If young male or castrated male and no evidence of scouring, particularly if on concentrate feed, then examination of urinary tract is essential.

- Check if recently castrated with bloodless castrator – incorrect technique may damage urethra.
- Check for urolithiasis.
- Examine prepuce for crystals adhering to preputial hairs or orifice. In young animals the penis cannot be extruded for examination.
- Palpate bladder for distension.
- Check for pain or discomfort when pressure is applied to pelvic inlet area.
- Check patency of urethra by careful pressure on bladder.

Note: A check on ability to urinate can be made by placing the animal in a clean dry pen for a couple of hours if this cannot be established by other methods. The extremely small diameter of the urethra makes catheterization impossible.

If urolithiasis occurs within a group, check water supply, and suitability of feed. Concentrates with a high phosphorus content are now thought to be the cause, although until recently high magnesium content was blamed. Some brands of ewe nuts specifically state that they should not be fed to lambs or rams.

Adult female

Although cystitis can occur at any time of the year and will cause tenesmus, most episodes of straining will be associated with active stages of the reproductive cycle.

During the mating period

- Check for traumatic vaginitis due to reactivation of adhesions resulting from damage at previous lambing.
- Check for infectious vulvovaginitis (examine rest of group and rams).

During mid-pregnancy

- Check for impacted mummified fetus
- Check for early abortion.

During pre-lambing and lambing period

- Check for impending abortion.
- Check for malpresentation.

- Check for incomplete dilatation of cervix.
- Check for torsion of uterus.
- Check for peri-anal herniation.

After lambing

- Check for retained lamb.
- Check for bruising or vaginal tears after traumatic lambing, or shepherd interference.

Note: Prolapse of the vagina and/or cervix will be an obvious cause of tenesmus and is dealt with in Chapter 4.

If no abnormality of the reproductive tract is detected, and the animal is not scouring, cystitis is a possibility, and a urine sample should be obtained for examination. This can be done by occluding the nostrils for a few seconds which stimulates urination, by catheterization, or if all else fails, by introducing a strange ram to the ewe which will usually react by urinating.

Adult male

- Check for urolithiasis (extrude penis and examine urethral appendage particularly).
- Check for penile trauma (urethral obstruction).
- Check for posthitis.
- Check for traumatic occlusion of the prepuce.

Note: Groups of rams may indulge in reproductive activity before joining, with mounting and insertion of the penis into the rectum of other members of the group. This can cause penile trauma and the possibility of rectal trauma.

12 Adult weight loss

Definition
Group weight loss
  Nutritional
  Parasitism
  Other chronic disease
Individual weight loss
  Tooth problems
  Other chronic disease, respiratory,
  digestive, neurological

Adult weight loss or poor body condition has always been a major problem in sheep keeping. However, the pattern and causes have changed over the years. In earlier periods when the industry was characterized by low input, low output systems, concurrent disease was likely to be the major cause. More recently, increased demand on inadequate inputs has become recognized as the most frequent source of problems.

Imbalance between nutritional demand and the supply of nutrients may be brought about by overt undersupply, or inability to ingest an adequate supply, or as a result of disease processes causing malabsorption, or interference with metabolic processes.

The masking effect of the fleece remains a major factor hindering detection of early weight loss in adult sheep. Frequently, by the time a problem is recognized, weight loss may have progressed to a degree which makes correction difficult. This occurs particularly and commonly during late pregnancy, when increasing nutritional demands and limited time available to deal with this are irreconcilable. The recent practice of winter shearing greatly facilitates control of body condition, where the management system allows this to be carried out.

A weight loss of 5% is recognized as indicating a problem in the human, if the loss takes place over a short time on normal inputs. This degree of monitoring is seldom available to the sheep keeper in the UK, as the variety of breeds and crosses have widely varying normal weight ranges. In countries where a more uniform sheep type predominates, regular weighing forms a vital management tool. This can be done by the use of individual 'indicator' groups.

The handling of individual sheep, and the application of the system of body condition scoring developed over recent years, allows a similar control of body condition to be maintained. It can be applied irrespective of breed, size or weight. It is important that the operator recognizes that its value lies in repeatability of results for the individual rather than between operators. The value can be much enhanced if a correlation is established between body condition scores and body weight for an individual breed or type, thus allowing a value to be placed on any change, i.e. a loss of one body score means the ewe has lost X kg. In the case of common types of crossbred ewe such as the mule or Welsh halfbred, one unit of condition score is equivalent to *approximately* 5 kg.

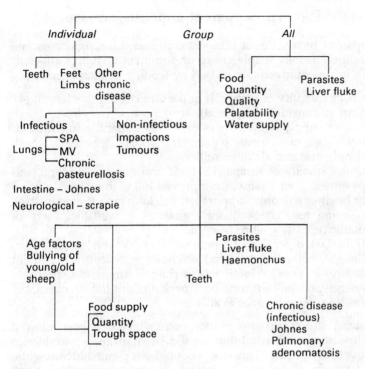

Figure 12.1 Adult loss of condition

In the investigation of any weight loss problem, the following aspects of the history are particularly relevant (see also Figure 12.1):

- Number affected – individual, many, whole group, all groups.
- Validity and extent of weight loss.
- Time scale of loss.
- Stage of cycle of nutritional demand.
- Recent management of nutrition.
- Any evidence of recent management changes, e.g. housing, change from hay to silage, etc.

Weight loss with apparent appetite increase

Apparent by continual hunger, continual bleating, or escape attempts, usually whole group or dominant members affected. This is almost invariably caused by feeding mismanagement.

- Check quantity of forage. If at pasture check grass length (4–6 cm is considered optimal). If at pasture in winter, check fodder supply (empty racks may mean quantity insufficient, full racks may mean palatability poor). If housed, check supply and actual consumption.
- Check quality of forage. Late autumn grass or undergrazed pasture is poor quality; unimproved hill with rushes, bracken or heather will only support low stocking rate. If hay or silage is being fed, check quality, analysis if available, stage of maturity, how well conserved.
- If in last 8 weeks of pregnancy, check concentrate feed. Bought-in feed – check price (cheap = nasty), ash content (>10% is poor). Home mix – check formulation, probable energy and protein content. Check amount fed, frequency of feeding, trough space available.

Note: At this stage of pregnancy, ewes which have been allowed to lose too much condition should be managed separately to allow extra feeding. This will produce better lamb birth weights, and possibly adequate colostrum, but it is impossible to put condition back on the ewes themselves.

Energy requirements of a 70 kg ewe rearing twins

In dry period	9.0 MJ/day
Flushing	15.0 MJ/day
Early pregnancy	15.0 MJ/day
Mid pregnancy	12.0 MJ/day
Late pregnancy	20.0 MJ/day
Early lactation	25.0–30.0 MJ/day
Mid lactation	15.0 MJ/day
Weaning	9.0 MJ/day

Note: If winter shorn, extra feed allowance is necessary – appetite will increase by at least 10% especially in cold weather.

Weight loss, appetite apparently normal, intake reduced

The most common cause of this pattern of weight loss is tooth problems. Incisor loss (broken mouth) will cause weight loss if grazing is short, but otherwise such sheep can remain in good condition, particularly if extra attention is given at times of nutritional stress. Molar problems are a very common and often unrecognized cause of weight loss (see also chapter 13 for more details). Shedding of temporary premolars is occasionally implicated, but most often, premature loosening of the lower first molar is the cause, and can occur as young as 2 years of age.

- Check incisor teeth.
- Check molar teeth (palpate through cheeks, and check mandibles for swellings).
- Check for lameness – painful foot lesion, e.g. footrot or foot abscess can lead to rapid weight loss, particularly in late pregnancy.

Weight loss with normal appetite and normal intake

Where *individual* animals are affected but the remainder of the group is in good bodily condition, the most likely cause is concurrent, usually chronic, disease.

- Check molar teeth as above.
- Check for Johnes disease – faeces sample for ZN stained smear. May need repeated sampling, or may not be identified until PME.
- Check for pulmonary adenomatosis (wheelbarrow test for excess pulmonary fluid). No other diagnostic test apart from PME.
- Check lungs for chronic pneumonia. Maedi-visna (MV) is an important cause of chronic lung lesions in other countries, but not in indigenous British sheep, although there is serological evidence of exposure to the virus where there has been contact with early imports of continental breeds, and a few clinical cases have now been seen.
- Check for cud spilling – long-term sufferers often are poor thrivers (see chapter 13).
- Check for early signs of scrapie – other neurological signs should be detectable, or an 'itch' reflex.

Other individual causes of weight loss such as tumours, liver abscess may only be diagnosed at PME.

Where *many sheep* are affected, the cause is likely to be either nutritional or concurrent disease, particularly parasitic.

If in mid-late pregnancy or lactation:
- Check quantity and quality of food, as above.

With ewes carrying multiple fetuses, it is almost impossible to prevent loss of condition in the last 3 weeks of gestation, when demand for energy is twice that for maintenance. The uterus and contents occupy up to 60% of available space so that appetite is much reduced. If the ewes entered mid pregnancy in good condition, the loss of condition can be accommodated. In early lactation the appetite increases dramatically, but with energy demand now being three times that of maintenance, weight loss is inevitable. A ewe maintaining triplets faces energy demands equivalent to the demands on a sow with 30 piglets!

Note: Rations which contain significant amounts of undegradable protein (UDP) actively encourage the metabolism of body fat to produce milk. Such diets should not be used for ewes of already poor bodily condition.

- Check also for age distribution – social pressures on young, old or less dominant members.
- Check trough space allowed.
- Check for chronic liver fluke – faeces sample. Number of eggs present is probably an indication of severity of infection, but even one is significant. Blood sample for liver enzymes – gamma glutamyl transferase (GGT) is indicator of chronic damage especially to bile ducts.
- Check for *Haemonchus* infection – anaemia and oedema associated with wasting. Chronic infection resembles malnutrition.

Where a *whole group* or *flock* is involved, nutritional factors are again the most likely cause, although parasitic problems should also be considered.

- Check whole feeding policy – roughage and concentrate quantity and quality.
- Check for owner inexperience.
- Check for owner with cash flow problem – unable to purchase sufficient feed.
- Check for overstocking – unreasonable expectation of capacity of land available.
- Check for mismanagement of winter shearing – failure to provide increased feed supply.
- Check cobalt and copper status. Although these trace elements are involved in failure to thrive in young animals, it would be uncommon for deficiency of these to cause weight loss in the adult – see chapter 9. Where copper availability is

reduced because of land improvement, weight loss in adult sheep may result.

Note: Where all feed inputs are home grown, the potential for accumulating deficiencies is aggravated. In this situation blood biochemistry is likely to be helpful, with samples taken from a minimum of six affected animals.

Samples required – heparinized, oxalate–fluoride and clotted blood. Check: glucose, AST, GDH, SDH, BHB, albumin, urea, Ca, Mg, inorganic P, copper, cobalt (vitamin B_{12}).

Weight loss, reduced appetite

Where *individual animals* are affected, the reduction in appetite is usually a result of concurrent disease affecting either the ability of the animal to obtain or ingest food, or the result of the disease process itself, particularly in the terminal stages.

- Check for lameness reducing mobility especially footrot, foot abscess, arthritis.
- Check for mouth lesions – see chapter 13.
- Check for gastrointestinal problem, e.g. rumen impaction, abomasal impaction, terminal Johnes disease.
- Check for sight problems – inability to see food.

    If in late pregnancy:
- Check for pregnancy toxaemia – typical symptoms of blindness, dullness and depression with evidence of large fetal load. Check blood sample for glucose, BHB, urea, albumin, calcium, magnesium.
- Check for imminent parturition – animals often have a reduced appetite immediately prepartum.

Where *many animals or whole groups* are affected, the cause is likely to be major interference with feed intake, or gross neglect of chronic disease such as liver fluke.

- Check for major outbreak of parasitic disease – liver fluke, haemonchosis – faeces samples for egg counts (see above).
- Check water supply – animals on a wet diet such as silage or roots need little extra water except when lactating. Animals on dry diets may drink several litres daily and considerably more when lactating. In such a case, deprivation for more than 24 h, e.g. frozen pipes, will have an effect on appetite.

- Check water palatability – contamination with chemicals, e.g. bitumen, creosote.
- Check food palatability – fungal spoilage of concentrates or forage, especially big bale silage, accidental contamination with chemicals, mistakes in mixing feed additives.

13 Mouth disorders

The presence of mouth lesions which cause difficulty in eating may often not become obvious until the animal loses flesh, or obvious signs of debility are present. This is an inevitable consequence of the inability of the shepherd in many commercial flocks to closely observe the grazing and ruminating behaviour of each individual animal. Where closer supervision is possible, for example in a small pedigree flock, mouth problems may be noted earlier, as a result of noticeable discomfort during eating or ruminating or by signs of quidding.

A sheep mouth gag and torch are essential pieces of equipment where any mouth examination is to be carried out. It is impossible to perform this examination adequately, except in the case of the young lamb, without these pieces of equipment because of the anatomy and temperament of the sheep. The distance to which the jaws can be opened is very limited, and it is impossible to examine the deeper recesses without an external light source. In addition, the clinician risks the injury or loss of fingers if these are inserted into the mouth without the protection of a gag.

Prolonged examination of the molar teeth causes considerable stress in the adult sheep, and the use of sedation or even general anaesthesia should be considered, particularly in the case of potentially valuable pedigree animals, where remedial dental work is likely to be required following the examination.

Before examination of the inside of the mouth of adult sheep, it is extremely helpful to palpate the mandibular rami where the presence of swellings will immediately indicate molar tooth problems, and to feel through the cheeks along the length of the molar teeth, where resentment to application of pressure will give a similar indication.

Although tooth problems in the adult animal dominate this subject, mouth problems of various types can affect all age groups.

The possibility of foot and mouth disease as a cause of excess salivation in association with sudden onset of lameness in a group of sheep should never be overlooked. Consult Divisional Veterinary Officer if in any doubt.

Neonatal lambs

Mouth problems should always be suspected in the young lamb which appears unable or unwilling to suck, although bright and alert in all other respects. There will rarely be external evidence that the mouth is the source of the problem.

Individual lamb affected

- Check for parturient trauma – separation of mandibular symphysis (poor lambing technique), swollen tongue.
- Check for cleft palate.
- Check for predator trauma – tongue tip missing.

Many young lambs affected

- Check for periodontal orf lesions.
Note: Severe orf lesions can be present in the mouth with little external evidence on the lips, within a few days of birth. This is particularly common in groups of artificially reared lambs.

Growing lambs

Individual lambs affected

- Check for trauma.

Many lambs affected

- Check for drenching gun injury.
These will usually be unilateral and similar in position in all affected animals, usually starting in the lateral buccal pouch and continuing towards the throat. Frequently there will be a characteristic putrid smell of necrotic tissue. If of several days' duration, the throat will be swollen, but in the early stages there will be no indication that the inability to eat is buccal in origin.

- Check for necrotic stomatitis.
Commissures show multiple necrotic lesions. May involve tongue, hard palate and cheeks. This condition is usually secondary to orf, or results from grazing abrasive weeds such as thistles or docks and brambles, and may be aggravated by trimming such weeds.

If in any doubt, check with Divisional Veterinary Officer about foot and mouth disease.

Adult sheep

Mouth disorders in older sheep fall generally into one of two categories. They may affect individual animals, producing signs which directly indicate that the mouth is the source of the problem. Alternatively, mouth lesions will only be identified

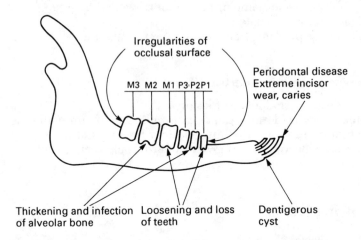

Figure 13.1 Common sites of tooth and jaw disorders in adult sheep

during investigation into a wider flock problem, usually weight loss, involving a number of animals. Figure 13.1 shows the common sites of tooth and jaw disorders.

Individual mouth problems

Excess salivation

- Check for trigeminal/facial paralysis – unilateral paralysis of ear, eyelid, facial muscles suggests listeriosis.
- Check for access to irritant plant or chemical poison.
- Check for throat lesions – inability to swallow saliva, drenching gun injury.

Cud spilling

- Check for molar tooth problem – eruption, impaction, looseness, loss.
- Check for breed – may be genetic predisposition.

- Check for ulceration or fibrosis of tongue – actinobacillosis.
- Possible actinobacillosis of oesophageal groove.

Swelling of mandible or submandibular region

In this category, molar tooth problems predominate. Almost invariably the first molar tooth is the first to become involved in any disease process. This is because this is the first permanent cheek tooth to erupt (at 3 months of age), whereas the adjoining permanent third premolar does not erupt until nearly 2 years of age.

In some cases, radiography of the jaws may be helpful to assess the extent of damage.

- Check for molar tooth problem.
- Check for actinomycosis of jaw.
- Check for actinobacillosis of cheek.
- Check for dentigerous cyst – incisor root area.
- Check for submandibular oedema – chronic fluke, haemonchosis.

Mouth disorders usually identified during investigation of a flock problem

There are two common conditions which usually affect significant numbers of animals or even whole groups. The client will consult not as to the presence, which is self evident on examination, but because of a high incidence or changing incidence, and the possible reasons for such changes. These conditions are incisor loss, and extreme incisor wear. Molar disease may also affect groups as well as more sporadic individual cases as described above, but these may not be recognized by the farmer.

There may not be a good correlation between body condition score and incisor tooth loss, except perhaps during winter feeding or in adverse environmental conditions, i.e. high hill farms. The relationship between body condition and molar tooth condition is more significant. Although farmers readily recognize incisor loss and cull for it (sometimes unnecessarily), molar disease which has much more serious consequences, may go largely unrecognized as previously mentioned.

Extreme incisor wear

- Check nutrition in early life – during tooth development.
- Check for evidence of fluorosis (bone samples required).
- Check geology – high sand content causing tooth wear.
- Check winter feeding – root feeding in sandy or frozen ground.

Note: True dental caries, with pitting of the incisors, does sometimes occur, and may be associated with high carbohydrate diets.

Periodontal disease, incisor tooth loss ('broken mouth')

- Check breed – incisor/dental pad apposition.
- Check feeding – big bale silage, self-feed silage.
- Check for use of feed blocks.

In spite of these suggestions, there is still no clear evidence as the the cause of this widespread condition which forces premature culling of many hill ewes. Trials involving moving sheep from unaffected flocks on to affected farms have shown that there is a definite individual farm incidence.

14 Lameness

Examination of the foot and limb
Lambs
   Trauma
   Joint infections
   Nutritional
Group adult lameness
   Mechanical
   Infections
Individual adult lameness
   Foot infections
   Non-infectious foot conditions
   Arthritis
   Acute mastitis

The individual lame sheep has long been assumed by the sheep keeper to be one of the inevitable burdens of the trade – like the poor always with us! This attitude is now changing with the realization that the lame sheep often presents welfare problems out of all proportion to the severity of the visible lesions. Quite apart from the concern of allowing unnecessary suffering, the modern sheep keeper accepts that any lameness, whatever the cause will give a significant loss of production. The clinician is therefore called on to diagnose and treat individual lame animals more frequently, and is no longer limited to giving assistance only in 'outbreaks' of lameness. In addition, the considerable value of stock rams or exotic breeds makes individual care worthwhile to the farmer.

The first decision the clinician must make is – does this clinical picture represent true lameness, i.e. the result of some patho-logical process in the foot, or in muscle, bone or joint? Or is it rather a case of locomotor disturbance, that is, the result of peripheral nerve or central nervous system lesions? Inevitably there will be some overlap with conditions discussed in Chapter 15 which covers neurological disease.

In some cases the differentiation may be obvious, for example a flock affected with chronic footrot, or cases of swayback in a known area or farm subject to copper deficiency. Generally, however, the veterinarian must rely on detailed examination of the history of each episode, combined with a knowledge of farm or area, and then an examination of the patient.

In young lambs, joint problems are a more important cause of lameness than foot lesions. In contrast, the vast majority of cases of lameness in adult sheep originate in the foot. An initial rapid examination may be made of the upper limb to eliminate obvious gross lesions such as fractures, but the main examina-tion should concentrate on the foot, returning to higher structures if the site of lameness is not found.

The possibility of foot and mouth disease should never be forgotten where there is sudden illness and lameness in a group of sheep. Consult Divisional Veterinary Officer if in doubt.

Examination of the foot

In some cases of acute foot lameness, the site of the lesion may be very difficult to locate. That the foot is indeed the site is simple enough to determine, when the classic signs of heat, pain and swelling are present. However, in the case of some penetrating foreign bodies, or the early stages of white line abscessation, careful searching is necessary to locate first the affected claw, then the actual site of the lesion. A good sharp knife, used carefully, together with a good pair of eyes are the most important diagnostic tools.

Note: Foot paring should always be done with great care. At the toe, the digital artery is easily cut if too much horn is removed, and this can lead to profuse haemorrhage immediately and chronic granuloma formation in the long term.

Examination of the upper limb

- Atrophy of muscles – indicates lameness of some duration.
- External injuries – may indicate possibility of fractures.
- Joint swellings – indicate septicaemic arthritis in the lamb, osteoarthritis in the aged animal.
- Other swellings – abscess, haematoma, trauma.
- Stance – abnormal may be to ease pain in foot, or may indicate nerve or tendon damage.

In the diagnosis of the cause of lameness, the age of the affected animal(s), the number affected, and the findings of the clinical examination will all narrow the field of possibilities.

Neonatal lambs

True lameness immediately after birth is not common, most cases resulting from trauma.

- Check for obstetric trauma (excessive traction) – fractures, dislocations, radial paralysis, bruised tendons.
- Check for fractures resulting from treading by dam or other ewes in confines of small pens.
- Check also for 'short' (contracted) tendons, usually bilateral affecting forelegs. Severe cases may be unable to stand, or walk on dorsal aspect of fetlocks.

Incoordination is common in young lambs, associated with faulty development of the nervous system, e.g. swayback, border disease, cerebellar hypoplasia. For more details see chapter 15.

Young lambs over 2 days of age

With the exception of trauma, incidents of lameness in young lambs will usually involve significant numbers of animals, either because the causes are management related, or infectious in origin in a group which is immunologically naive. Joint lesions are likely to be more common that foot lesions in this group.

Individual lamb, sudden lameness

- Check for trauma – fractured leg (trodden on by adult sheep).
- Check for foreign body – thorns easily penetrate the soft horn.
- Check claws of affected leg for abscessation. Abscesses occasionally develop within a few days of birth, and usually affect one digit only.

Note: Occasional outbreaks of a probable hereditary condition known as 'redfoot' are seen, particularly in Scottish blackface lambs, although rarely other breeds may be affected. This is a defect of the skin epithelium which leads to horn loss, infection and progressive lameness. Mouth and eye lesions may also be present.

Many lambs affected

The most common causes of lameness are:

Joint infections
    neonatal septicaemia/polyarthritis
    tick pyaemia
Foot infections
    footrot
    scald
Nutritional myopathy
    selenium/vitamin E deficiency
Nutritional osteopathy
    osteoporosis, rickets

- Check for neonatal polyarthritis. Usually affects several joints in more than one limb, but is rarely bilaterally symmetrical. The knee and stifle are most commonly affected. In some cases, joint distension may be obvious, but in other cases severe lameness may exist with minimal detectable joint abnormality.

A variety of bacteria are found in these cases – *Staphylococcus, Streptococcus*, Coliforms, *Actinomyces (Corynebacterium) pyogenes, Fusobacterium necrophorum, Erysipelothrix rhusiopathiae*.

These cannot be differentiated on clinical grounds. If lambs do not respond to treatment, samples of joint fluid from untreated cases should be submitted for bacteriological examination. Check also for concurrent navel infection. These conditions are usually associated with poor hygiene in the lambing pens, or application of dirty castrating or tailing rings. See also chapter 8, perinatal lamb losses.

- If lambs are lame from about 2 weeks onwards with swollen joints, and are on rough or tick-infested pasture, check for tick pyaemia – this results from *Staph. aureus* infection gaining access to joints in lambs suffering from concurrent tick-borne fever which lowers resistance to infection. Abscesses may be present in other parts of the body, e.g. spinal cord, liver. If bacteriological investigation shows bacteria other than *Staph. aureus* present, the case is likely to be one of neonatal polyarthritis rather than tick pyaemia.
- Check for scald or early footrot lesions – typical moist lesions in cleft, non-progressive if scald, progresses to separation of sole from heel if footrot present. Footrot is less common in young lambs than older ones, but can occur. See later for more details.
- If lambs are stiff, unable to move, or collapse on being driven, check for nutritional myopathy (white muscle disease, vitamin E/selenium deficiency). This disease picture can be confused with neonatal polyarthritis – careful examination should be made of the joints. Often affects fast growing lambs, and stiffness is characteristically seen in the shoulder muscles which may atrophy if successful treatment is not given quickly. The condition is often very painful to the affected lamb, and it may be unable to rise from lateral recumbency. Check creatinine kinase (CK) concentration (serum or plasma sample required). Should be taken early in course of disease as concentration falls after a few days. >1000 i.u./ml is significant. Check rest of group (six minimum) for GSH-Px – heparinized samples required.
- Check if creep containing monensin is being fed – check very carefully inclusion rate (normally 15 ppm). Monensin poisoning can closely resemble nutritional myopathy. May also be some reluctance to eat as monensin is unpalatable.

Growing lambs (Figures 14.1 and 14.2)

Many of the conditions affecting very young lambs will continue to affect this older age group. In addition, lesions acquired in early life in a mild undetected form may become apparent. Nutritional myopathies and osteopathies may be more apparent during this growing phase. With increasing age, hoof conformation and overgrowth will become of more significance as contributory factors in the development of true foot rot.

- Check for foot lesions – footrot, scald, soreness as result of fertilizer application with lambs remaining on field.
- Check for foreign body especially thorns.
- Check for polyarthritis caused by *Erysipelothrix rhusiopathiae* (*insidiosa*), or *Chlamydia psittaci*. Lambs are 'poor thrivers' with marked stiffness or lameness and muscle wastage especially in upper hind limbs. These two conditions cannot be distinguished clinically. Both cause insidious joint damage *without* much obvious joint swelling. Careful palpation is required to detect affected joints although these become more obvious as the disease progresses because of muscle wastage. Collect sample of joint fluid for stained smear and bacteriological examination (may be no growth if antibiotic treatment has been given). Blood sample for serology. This is very helpful in erysipelas cases where a high titre is significant. Check for possible contact with pigs, or use of old pig pens for young lambs.

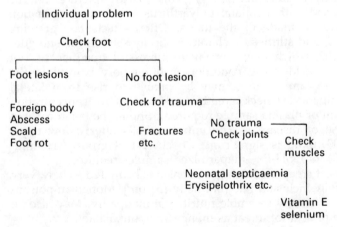

Figure 14.1 Lameness in growing lambs – individual problem

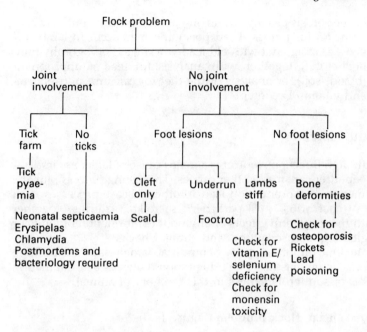

NB Post-dipping lameness

Figure 14.2 Lameness in growing lambs – flock problem

With *Chlamydia,* care in interpretation is needed if the flock is affected with EAE. Paired samples are helpful to indicate rising titre.

- Check also for chronic effects of neonatal polyarthritis (pus present in joints which may burst).
- Check for nutritional myopathy as above.
- Check inclusion rate of monensin if used.
- Check for post dipping lameness (*E. rhusiopathiae*) – feet are hot and swollen, sheep may be pyrexic with septicaemia and polyarthritis. History and clinical signs should be diagnostic. Serology is not helpful. It may be possible to isolate the organism from blood or exudate from lesions.
- If lambs have leg deformities, osteoporosis or stunted growth, check for rickets, nutritional osteopathy (bent leg, double scalp), or for lead poisoning. All of these conditions should be considered in the absence of another diagnosis. Rickets may occur in fast growing lambs reared indoors away from sunlight.

- Osteoporosis usually occurs on poor hill pasture, but may also occur on lush grass. Lead poisoning may occur in lambs on ewes grazing land with old lead workings. Radiography may be helpful, together with analysis for lead if appropriate (blood, soil), or analysis of the diet for calcium, phosphorus and vitamin D content.

Adult sheep

Although infectious footrot is a major cause of lameness in adult sheep, there are many other causes. The ageing process plus the demands of reproduction lead to other disease processes such as osteoarthritis, post-parturient sacroiliac arthritis, together with the long-term effects of any poor conformation of joints or digits, e.g. corkscrew toe, and straight hocks.
Note: One important cause of hindlimb lameness in the lactating ewe is acute mastitis. The udder should always be examined in cases of sudden lameness in this category of animal.

Lame sheep, flock problem (Figure 14.3)

Do not forget the possibility of foot and mouth disease where sudden flock lameness is accompanied by systemic illness.

The common types of flock lameness are scald, footrot, white line disease, soil balling and post-dipping lameness. In each case the foot lesions are diagnostic.

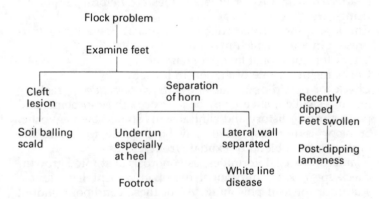

NB Foot and mouth disease

Figure 14.3 Lameness in adult sheep – flock problem

Scald
Scald is limited to the cleft, with moist raw areas on the axial surfaces of the claws which cause considerable pain, although the sheep is able to run when necessary. This infection, which is caused by *Fusobacterium necrophorum* or non-invasive *Bacteroides nodosus*, never progresses beyond the foot cleft.

● If housed, check for dirty or damp bedding.
● If outside, check for dirty or muddy areas around feeding or drinking troughs.

Footrot
Footrot is still the most common flock problem, since repeated infection does not induce a useful immune response. Carrier sheep are very common, and detailed examination of all feet is necessary to detect all such animals, although in many cases an obvious deformity of the hoof or horn is present.

Caused by the synergistic action of *Bacteroides nodosus* and *Fusobacterium necrophorum*. There are a number of strains of *B. nodosus* which vary in invasiveness. Early lesions are similar to scald, but progress to separation of the sole usually beginning at the heels. Invasive strains cause separation right across the sole and up the wall of the hoof. More than one foot may be affected at the same time.

● Check for characteristic foul smell.
● Isolation of *B. nodosus* and typing of strain can be done, but is rarely required. Special transport medium is needed.
● Check all feet carefully for carrier animals – horn deformity may indicate underlying pockets of infection.

White line disease
White line disease is a common cause of lameness in individual sheep, but may also be sufficiently widespread to be considered a flock problem. Separation of the lateral hoof wall occurs at the position of the white line. The pocket thus formed becomes impacted with mud and grit, and may lead to the development of a foot abscess. The cause is unknown, although there is a suggestion that zinc deficiency may be implicated.

Soil balling
Soil balling (packing of cleft with a hard mixture of grass and mud) is extremely common in lowland flocks on lush grass, particularly in late autumn. The skin of the cleft becomes sore as a result of the hard grass-mud mixture which becomes

trapped between the claws. Little can be done to prevent this, except for keeping sheep on well-grazed pasture at this time.

A similar condition can develop in housed sheep where a 'shoe' of matted bedding and faeces can cause similar discomfort.

Post-dipping lameness

Post-dipping lameness is associated with dipping in dirty or contaminated dips. A few days after dipping the feet are hot and swollen, sheep may be pyrexic with septicaemia and polyarthritis. History and clinical signs should be diagnostic. Serology is not helpful. It may be possible to isolate the organism (*E. rhusiopathiae*) from blood or exudate from lesions.

- Check for hygiene around dipping pens.
- Check for gross contamination of dip.
- Check for re-use of dip without addition of bacteriostat.

Individual lame sheep (Figure 14.4)

All the previous conditions may occur within a flock at a low incidence. In addition there are a variety of important causes of lameness which may affect individual sheep. The most common are: foot abscess, white line disease, foreign body, trauma, granuloma, interdigital fibroma, impacted interdigital sebaceous gland, laminitis, poor conformation, e.g. corkscrew claws, osteoarthritis and mastitis.

As stated previously, a very careful examination of the foot should be carried out. Whilst some lesions will be obvious, others may not.

Acute lameness

- Check for foot abscess.

Heat and pain will be present in the affected claw, but swelling may not appear until late in the process, by which time irreparable damage may have been done. The affected claw should be carefully pared and any tracks followed, particularly those running up the wall of the hoof. Often the horn is so hard that paring is impossible. Poulticing for 24 h softens the horn making this much easier. Great care should be taken to avoid causing haemorrhage which may lead to long-term granuloma problems.

Foot abscess usually follows one of two courses.

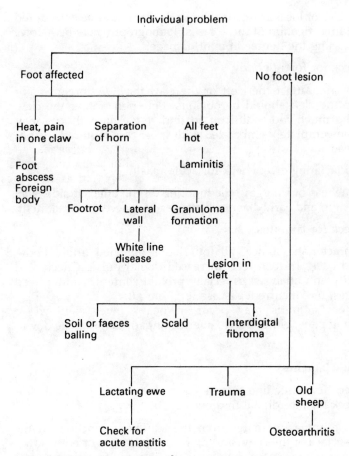

Figure 14.4 Lameness in adult sheep – individual problem

(1) Pus formation remains superficial, running up under the lateral wall of the claw, eventually bursting at the coronet if not relieved before. After drainage of pus, the lateral wall separates and can be pared away leaving no permanent damage.

(2) Deep infection of the claw takes place, with the pedal joint becoming involved. Swelling of the foot occurs, and sinuses discharging pus appear at several points around the coronary band including axially within the cleft. A septic arthritis quickly becomes established. Heavy rams seem particularly prone to this type.

Note: Use of local or regional anaesthesia should be considered in the investigation of these cases. Radiography may be helpful in assessing the degree of joint damage.

● Check for foreign body.

This may affect the cleft or the claw itself. A foreign body within the cleft should be obvious. One penetrating the claw may be much more difficult to find, e.g. sharp thorns may become completely embedded with great care required to spot the head.

● In a lactating ewe, check for acute mastitis.

Lameness or dragging the hind leg on the affected side is an early sign, and early diagnosis may lead to successful treatment.

● Check for laminitis.

Characteristic stance, all four limbs bunched under body, arched back, heat in feet, increased digital pulse. Check feed quantity and analysis, especially protein content, sudden feed changes, or concurrent disease, e.g. metritis.
Note: Laminitis may occur in heavy ewes confined to fostering pens, either due to overfeeding, or failure to lie down.

Chronic lameness

● Check for white line disease – see above.
● Check for interdigital fibroma.

The fibroma originates from the skin/horn junction on the axial surface of the claw, and may arise from one or both claws, occupying the space between the claws. Excoriation and infection of the fibroma are common, leading to 'pinching' and lameness. It is particularly common in heavy Suffolks and may have a genetic predisposition.

● Check for impaction of the interdigital sebaceous gland.

This is not usually a cause of serious lameness, but occasionally the swelling forces the claws apart allowing excoriation of the skin of the cleft.

● Check for chronic granuloma formation.

Damage to the sensitive laminae by overparing, foot abscess or foreign body can lead to granuloma formation and failure of the horn to completely repair. Often the horn grows to hide the

granuloma, but careful paring will re-expose it. Check also for pockets of chronic footrot infection in this type of lesion.
Note: If the granuloma is cut, profuse haemorrhage will result.

● In old sheep, check for osteoarthritis.

This can affect one or more limbs, front or hind. In the forelimb, the usual site is the elbow. Palpation will reveal bony enlargement of the joint with restricted flexion. It is usually, although not always, bilateral. Severe lesions lead to a character-istic 'restricted' movement of the front legs when walking, and to 'paddling' movements resting alternate limbs when standing. In the hind limbs, the sacroiliac joints and hip joints may be affected, causing incoordination rather than actual lameness.

● Check for abnormalities of conformation.

Abnormalities of claw structure, e.g. corkscrew claws, or overgrowth of horn may predispose to lameness by allowing impaction with mud, or placing abnormal stresses on joints. Similarly abnormalities such as excessively straight hocks or extreme sloping pasterns may induce stresses leading to eventual lameness. A hereditary component may be involved in all these conditions.

15 Changed behaviour/neurological dysfunction

Common types of neurological disease
Neurological examination
Lambs
   Congenital
   Trauma
   Metabolic/nutritional
   Infection
Growing lambs
   Metabolic/nutritional
   Trauma
   Infection
   Space-occupying lesions
   Toxins
Adults
   Metabolic/nutritional
   Infection
   Space-occupying lesions
   Trauma
   Degenerative disease
   Toxins

There exists a wide range of conditions resulting from dysfunction somewhere within the nervous system which have either an effect on the behaviour of the animal, or cause alterations in the ability to stand or walk normally. Depending upon the site and nature of the problem, the animal may be mentally normal, depressed or hyperexcitable, and may exhibit other signs ranging from slight incoordination to total collapse. In some cases there is an obvious macroscopic lesion centrally or peripherally (for example an abscess in the brain or traumatic injury to a nerve), or microscopic lesions may be present (for example in listeriosis or scrapie). In other cases the problem results from alterations in constituents of the blood (for example hypocalcaemia, hypomagnesaemia) which affect neurological function without the presence of any macroscopic or microscopic lesion.

Whilst major changes will be immediately apparent to the sheep keeper, minor changes may only become noticeable during normal shepherding activities such as rounding up with dogs, driving, etc. A knowledge of individual behaviour within the flock (leadership, dominance, awkwardness, etc.) will need to be combined with observations of response to external stimuli in order to reach an overall assessment of behaviour as being normal or abnormal. To the competent shepherd it is often minor changes in behaviour or response to stimuli which indicate the early onset of many diseases.

The clinician must determine whether any behavioural change observed is in fact non-physiological. Change in behaviour can be profound, but still be a normal physiological response. For example, some normal animals will adopt a recumbent or freezing posture merely in response to cornering or catching. A neonatal lamb may not show 'flight' behaviour simply because it has failed to bond with a ewe. A parturient ewe may not show flight because a lambing site has been selected, and perhaps most obviously, the ewe with a newborn lamb will show fight and not flight behaviour to possible predators. It is also important to recognize an inability to react because of some gross physical disability such as severe lameness or arthritis.

Common types of neurological disease

A multiplicity of diseases have, not surprisingly, effects upon the normal function of the central and peripheral nervous system, but for common conditions of sheep these can be broken down into a small number of groups according to the type of disease process:

- developmental, e.g. congenital malformations,
- infections
    viruses
    bacteria
    parasites
- metabolic and nutritional,
- toxins,
- injuries,
- peripheral nerve or muscle abnormalities.

In many cases, diseases are limited to, or are most common in, a particular age group. Speed of onset and progression of the signs are also important indicators in diagnosis (Table 15.1). Where the cause of a particular problem is not immediately clear, a neurological examination should be carried out in a logical progression, which should enable the clinician to answer the questions – where is the lesion? (brain, spinal cord, peripheral nerves or muscles?) and what is likely to be causing it? The following outline summarizes the most useful neurological tests which can be applied to sheep. Notes should be made of the results of all observations, since it is likely that a diagnosis can only be made by an overall assessment.

Table 15.1 Timescale of onset of signs as guide to diagnosis in neurological disease

Time taken for signs to develop	Disease	Diagnostic aids
Immediate	Cervical injury	Groups of rams fighting
Minutes	Hypomagnesaemia	Response to treatment
Minutes–hours	Hypocalcaemia	Response to treatment
Hours	CCN	Opisthotonus, strabismus, Response to treatment
Hours–days	Pregnancy toxaemia	Urine (ketones) Blood (glucose, BHB)
Hours–days	Louping ill	Tick area, time of tick activity
Hours–day	Listeriosis	Silage feeding (poor quality) Scour, possible abortions
Days	Spinal abscess	Progressive, raised total WBC, Crossover
Weeks–months	Scrapie	Usually >2 years of age Often excessive pruritis
Weeks–months	Gid	Usually <2 years of age. Gradual onset, progressive

Routine for neurological examination

(1) Assess state of consciousness:
Hyperexcited – increased responsiveness, nervousness, fits,
Alert – normal demeanour,
Depressed – reduced responsiveness,
Stupor – difficulty arousing,
Comatose – cannot be aroused.
(2) Assess for any abnormal behaviour:
Circling,
Head pressing,
Aimless wandering,
Turning in one direction,
Becoming stuck in corners.
(3) Assess gait:
Dysmetria (hypometria/hypermetria),
Ataxia,
Paresis,
Paraplegia.
(4) Test postural reactions – these help to identify minor deficits
or differences between the two sides of the body. Blindfold-
ing accentuates abnormalities:
Head position,
Wheelbarrow test,
Hemistanding,
Hemiwalking,
Hopping,
Proprioceptive positioning (foot position).
(5) Test muscle tone (normal, flaccid, spastic), and pedal and
panniculus reflex.
(6) Examine head:
Menace test,
Blindfold each eye in turn and assess vision,
Strabismus,
Abnormal nystagmus,
Cheek sensation,
Ear and eyelid position.
(7) Take blood samples if necessary.
Blood sampling – neutrophils may show increase, or may be
'crossover' (more polymorphs than lymphocytes) if there is
a septic focus, but not necessarily if the lesion is well
circumscribed.
(8) Take CSF sample if necessary (under general anaesthesia
from the atlanto-occipital space, with head flexed – site is in

midline slightly proximal to a line joining anterior borders of wings of atlas, or under local anaesthesia from the lumbosacral space).

Examination of CSF
This may be helpful where a diagnosis is in doubt. Normal CSF is clear, colourless and contains no clots.

Abnormalities

- Yellow colour indicates haemorrhage or jaundice.
- Turbidity indicates increased cell content – infection.
- Blood indicates faulty technique, haemorrhage or trauma.
- Clots show increased fibrinogen or protein.
- Increased protein or lowered glucose content (use urine sticks to test) may indicate infection.
- CSF can also be used for calcium and magnesium estimation, and for bacterial culture.

Some common neurological abnormalities seen in sheep, related to the possible site of lesion

Cerebrum	behavioural change
	stupor, coma
	reduced menace response
	head aversion
	unilateral proprioceptive defects (contralateral)
Cerebellum	ataxia
	dysmetria
	nystagmus
	head tremor
	head tilt
	eyes fix but no menace response
	unilateral proprioceptive defects (ipsilateral)
Cranial nerves	
Oculomotor III	pupil asymmetry
	strabismus
Trochlear IV	strabismus
Trigeminal V	decreased facial sensation
	lower jaw paralysis
Abducens VI	strabismus

Facial VII	drooping ear, eyelid, lips
Vestibulocochlear VIII	nystagmus
Glossopharyngeal IX ⎫ Vagus X ⎬ Accessory XI ⎭	dysphagia
Hypoglossal XII	tongue paralysis
Spinal cord	paresis, paralysis
Proximal to T2	recumbent, unable to sit up
Distal to T2	recumbent, uses forelimbs
T1 to S1	panniculus reflex affected
Peripheral nerves	unilateral paresis, paralysis.

Note: This is by no means an exhaustive list. Some signs are more reliable than others, and transmitted pressure effects of a large lesion may cause anomalous signs.

Common diseases in which neurological abnormalities are seen

In all age groups, trauma to either the head, back or extremities is an obvious cause of neurological problems. In addition, three common procedures, if carried out incorrectly or carelessly can cause damage.

(1) Injection close to a major nerve, e.g. the sciatic, can cause muscle paralysis.
(2) Injection with contaminated needle or drug can lead to abscess formation which can involve adjacent nerves.
(3) Drenching gun injuries in the pharynx cause sepsis which can easily spread to the high cervical spinal cord.

Other common neurological problems can be categorized according to the age group most often affected, and often by the speed of onset and progression of symptoms.

Neonatal lambs

In the newborn lamb, neurological abnormalities fall into two main categories – congenital abnormalities and those due to dystocia (see Figure 15.1). The commonest are a result of:

● trauma during birth (anoxia, subcranial haemorrhage, peripheral nerve damage),

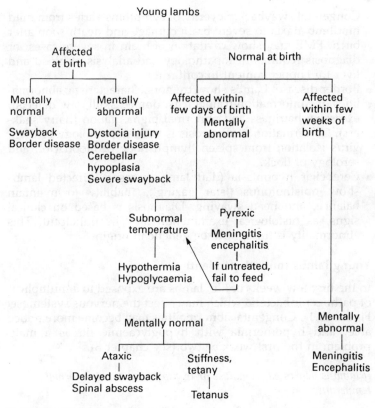

Figure 15.1 Diagnosis of neurological disease in young lambs

- hypoglycaemia as a result of failure to suck. Lambs which have suffered dystocia, particularly oversized lambs, are very susceptible,
- congenital swayback,
- border disease infection in early pregnancy,
- cerebellar hypoplasia.

Lambs unable to stand, or ataxic at birth
Check for:

- History of dystocia, especially if large lamb. Hypoxia or subcranial haemorrhage may affect ability of lamb to stand and suck. These lambs are particularly susceptible to hypothermia/hypoglycaemia. Prolonged dystocia may also cause peripheral nerve damage, e.g. radial paralysis.

- Congenital swayback. Severity of symptoms varies from mild hindlimb ataxia to severe brain damage and death soon after birth. PME may show cavitation of brain in severe cases, or diagnosis requires histopathology and analysis of blood and liver for copper content to confirm.
- Border disease. Lambs show tremors, characteristic abnormalities of conformation (camel legs, domed skull, jaw defects), excessive hairiness and abnormal pigmentation (hairy shakers). Confirmation of diagnosis is by histopathology of CNS, virus isolation from spleen, lymph node or blood clot, and serology of flock.
- Cerebellar hypoplasia (daft lamb disease). Affected lambs show opisthotonus ('star gazing'), inability to maintain balance, and head swaying. Diagnosis is based on clinical signs, as histological examination may be unhelpful. This abnormality is thought to be genetic in origin.

Young lambs (milk dependent)

In the first few weeks of life, lambs are exposed to a multiplicity of pathogenic bacteria which may affect the nervous system (see Figure 15.1). Congenital abnormalities may become more noticeable, and hypothermia with hypoglycaemic fits is a major problem in the first week or two (see chapter 8).

If lamb is depressed, comatose or in fits, and has a subnormal temperature.

- Suspect hypothermia. Should respond to intraperitoneal or intravenous glucose administration followed by warming. If it does not recover, PME shows brown fat stores depleted (see chapter 8).

If lamb is mentally normal, with incoordination or paresis of hindlegs

Check for the following.

- Spinal abscess – common site is C7–T2. Infection may also spread forwards from docking wounds or from infected navel. Symptoms are progressive, beginning with slight ataxia which usually worsens over a few days to complete hindlimb paralysis. May be response to antibiotics if treated early enough.
- In tick area, tick pyaemia – multiple abscesses from which *Staph. aureus* is isolated.
- Delayed swayback. This may also be progressive, but not

usually to total paralysis of hindlegs – swaying at hocks when made to run is most characteristic. There is no response to antibiotic therapy. Diagnosis requires blood or liver for copper estimation, and may require histological examination for confirmation.

If lamb is mentally abnormal, pyrexic, stiff neck, progressing to opisthotonus

Check for the following.

- Meningitis/encephalitis. This is often associated with other conditions resulting from poor hygiene at lambing – navel infections, septicaemia, enteritis, polyarthritis.
- *L. monocytogenes* – may occasionally cause neurological signs in young lambs, although septicaemia is more commonly associated with this organism in this age group.

If lamb shows generalized stiffness, hyperaesthesia and spasms.

- Suspect tetanus – check vaccination history, recent wounds, e.g. tailing, castration.

Growing lambs (Figure 15.2)

In this age group, the speed of onset of signs may be helpful in reaching a diagnosis.

Sudden onset of signs

- If animal is recumbent, blind, showing strabismus and opisthotonus, suspect cerebrocortical necrosis (CCN). Response to therapy (thiamine IV) is the best pointer to correct diagnosis in an early case. Blood sample (heparinized) can be taken for transketolase estimation (this is a specific test for CCN), and faecal sample for thiaminase estimation. In a dead animal rumen contents for thiaminase, and examination of the brain (yellow discoloration of the cerebral hemispheres and fluorescence under UV light) will confirm.
- If animal shows cerebellar signs (tremor, dysmetria and nystagmus), often with rapid deterioration, suspect cerebellar gid cyst or possibly abscess (see below).
- If in tick area, check for louping ill – incoordination progressing to paralysis, coma and death in 1–2 days. Samples required from live animal are heparinized blood and CSF, from dead animal remove brain, put small sample

of brain stem into 50% glycerol saline for virus isolation and rest into formol saline for histology.

- If lamb has been losing condition, drinking excess and develops fits suspect nephrosis. Take blood sample for creatinine and urea estimation to confirm. Where lambs with pulpy kidney are seen alive, these may exhibit fits before death occurs.
- If one of a group of young rams shows sudden onset of ataxia but is mentally alert, suspect damage to cervical vertebrae (cervical subluxation) as result of fighting. Radiography may be helpful in the case of a valuable animal. Similar signs may also result from a rapidly developing cervical spinal abscess. Check white blood cells (WBC) and differential count.

Gradual onset of signs

- If hindlimb ataxia is present, check for delayed swayback or spinal abscess as above.
- In area of high lead content, check for chronic lead poisoning. Animals show hindlimb ataxia, and there is often an associated osteoporosis with bone fractures.
- If animal shows visual deficits, postural deficits, circling or head aversion, check for space-occupying lesion in cerebral cortex (on opposite side from that showing deficits). The commonest causes are brain abscesses and *Taenia multiceps* (*Coenurus cerebralis*) cysts ('gid', 'sturdy').

Differentiation between these may be difficult unless there is a history of gid on the farm. Blood sampling may be helpful (a raised WBC count or crossover may indicate an abscess), and there may be response to vigorous antibiotic therapy in the case of an abscess. In advanced cases of gid there is often detectable skull softening present (but not necessarily on the side of the cyst).

Adults (Figure 15.3)

Sudden onset, individual animals affected

- If an adult ram in group of rams shows ataxia or paresis, suspect cervical trauma or concussion from fighting.
- If animal shows signs of space-occupying lesion in cerebrum or cerebellum suspect 'gid' (rarely affects those over 2 years old) or abscess. See above.

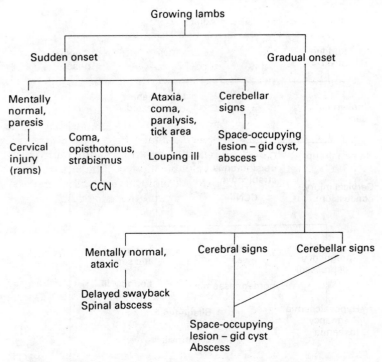

Figure 15.2 Diagnosis of neurological disease in growing lambs

- If animal shows collapse, blindness, strabismus and opisthotonus, suspect CCN. See above.

Sudden onset, many animals affected

- If are ewes in late pregnancy, suspect hypocalcaemia. Animals show incoordination followed by recumbency and death within a few hours. Response to treatment is the best confirmation of diagnosis, but take clotted blood sample pretreatment in case of no response. Hypocalcaemia often follows stress such as gathering, housing, vaccination, bad weather. It may co-exist with pregnancy toxaemia.
- If ewes are in poor condition in late pregnancy, suspect pregnancy toxaemia. Depression, loss of appetite, and apparent blindness are followed by recumbency within a few days. Clinical signs, body condition and probable high fetal load all point to the diagnosis which may be confirmed by showing ketones in urine, high BHB and low glucose concentrations in blood samples (take oxalate fluoride (OxF) and clotted

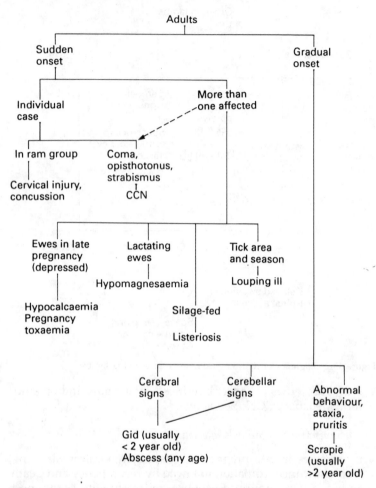

Figure 15.3 Diagnosis of neurological disease in adult sheep

samples). Liver enzymes are also raised. If the animal dies, PME shows a pale fatty liver.

If there is a flock problem, nutrition in the last 8 weeks of pregnancy should be investigated.

- If ewes are suckling lambs on good pasture, suspect hypomagnesaemia. Animals show trembling, hyperaesthesia, collapse and tetany. Symptoms worsen over minutes rather than hours. Some will respond to treatment, but others may die

during treatment. Take blood sample (clotted) from live animal, CSF or aqueous humour from dead animal.
- If animals are silage fed, show profound depression, circling or facial paralysis with protrusion of tongue and drooling of saliva, suspect listeriosis. Many affected animals die, in spite of treatment, within a few days. Diagnosis is by characteristic histology of brain, plus isolation of organism (this may take time as it is slow to grow).

   Check silage quality, soil contamination, fermentation (pH of good silage should be below 5), and method of feeding – uneaten silage should be cleared daily to prevent secondary fermentation. If there is a particular problem, check if sheep grazed silage fields before making – faecal excretion can contaminate grass. The organism is thought to gain access to the brain via wounds in the mouth or at teething from where it travels along nerve fibres.

- Although rare, the possibility of botulism should be borne in mind (badly made big bale silage may be responsible). Signs are muscular weakness progressing to flaccid paralysis.
- If in tick area, check for louping ill – see above.

Gradual onset of symptoms, slow progression

Individuals affected:

- If animal shows visual deficits, postural deficits, circling or head aversion, or cerebellar signs, check for 'gid' – see above. Gid is rarely seen in animals more than 2 years old.
- If animal shows incoordination, abnormal behaviour, loss of weight, excitement, excessive scratching, or any combination of these signs, suspect scrapie. There is no diagnostic test in the live animal. Cases usually deteriorate over a period of weeks. Positive diagnosis requires brain histology. If in breeding flock, particularly pedigree, investigate familial relationships and point out implications. Scrapie is rare in animals less than 2 years old.

Note: Cases of scrapie in younger animals, with quite rapid onset of signs and deterioration appear to be occurring more commonly.

- If animal shows dullness and twitching of muscles, consider uraemia – blood sample for urea and creatinine estimation.
- In a lactating ewe rearing twins or triplets, if function of both forelegs is lost with muscle atrophy, suspect 'kangaroo gait'.

Table 15.2 Postmortem diagnosis of some neurological diseases

Disease	Gross pathology	Microbiology	Biochemistry	Parasitology	Histopathology
Swayback	± Cavitation	–	Low Cu	–	+
Border disease	± Characteristic lambs	+ Virus isolation	–	–	+
Cerebellar hypoplasia	±	–	–	–	±?
Hypothermia/ hypoglycaemia	± Oedema of extremities	–	Low glucose	–	–
Encephalitis/ meningitis	+	+	–	–	+
Abscess	+	+	–	–	+
CCN	+ Yellowing of cerebrum	–	Raised TK	–	+
Louping ill	–	+ Virus isolation	–	–	+
Gid	+	–	–	+	No inflammatory reaction
Hypocalcaemia	–	–	Low Ca[Mg]	–	–
Hypomagnesaemia	–	–	Low Mg	–	–
Pregnancy toxaemia	+ Fatty liver	–	Ketones in urine Low glucose Raised BHB	–	+ (Liver)
Listeriosis	–	+	–	–	+
Scrapie	–	–	–	–	+

The cause of this peculiar condition is unknown but it is reversible, animals returning to normal after weaning.

Many animals affected:

- If animals are grazing ryegrass pasture and show tremors, knuckling of extremities and collapse, but recover after rest, consider mycotoxicosis ('migram', ryegrass staggers). This results from a toxin produced in fungi which parasitizes the seeds of ryegrass.

Table 15.2 summarizes the postmortem diagnosis of the neurological diseases mentioned here.

16 Eye disorders/ visual defects

Congenital
Infections
Trauma
Metabolic/nutritional
Degenerative
Space-occupying lesions

Defects in vision can arise from a wide variety of conditions, ranging from corneal disease at one extreme to a space-occupying lesion in the visual cortex at the other.

Diagnosis of the cause of impaired vision must start with the establishment of the site and nature of such impairment. In the case of corneal involvement, these may be obvious. In other cases, however, where the lesion is not obvious, it is essential that a full history is obtained and clinical examination is carried out.

Age, number affected, stage of reproductive cycle, general behaviour patterns, response to stimuli, body score in comparison with contemporaries, may all give vital indications of the presence of a disease which has its origins centrally, rather than in the orbit, but manifests itself primarily as a defect in vision.

The clinical examination should begin with an examination of the eyelids and superficial structures of the eye (Figure 16.1). Use of an ophthalmoscope will assist in the diagnosis of bright blindness (retinal atrophy), but oedema of the optic disc does not seem to be a feature of increased intracranial pressure in the sheep.

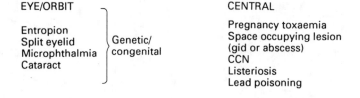

EYE/ORBIT

Entropion
Split eyelid   Genetic/
Microphthalmia   congenital
Cataract

CENTRAL

Pregnancy toxaemia
Space occupying lesion
(gid or abscess)
CCN
Listeriosis
Lead poisoning

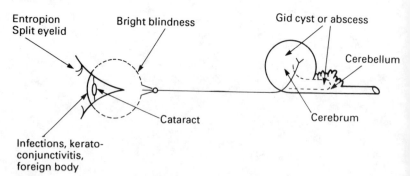

Entropion
Split eyelid   Bright blindness   Gid cyst or abscess

Cerebellum

Cataract   Cerebrum

Infections, kerato-
conjunctivitis,
foreign body

Figure 16.1 Site of lesion in diseases affecting the eye or vision

The integrity of the visual pathways can be tested with the menace (blink) test. Where lesions causing visual defects are present in the brain, other neurological signs or deficits will usually be present. See chapter 15 for more details.

The age of the patient(s) and the number affected will be the first guide to a possible diagnosis.

Neonatal lambs

Check for congenital or genetic factors.

• Entropion leads to a secondary keratitis if treatment is delayed. This condition now affects many breeds and crosses.

Note: Almost all cases of young lambs which are presented by the farmer as suffering from 'New Forest disease' will in fact be corneal infection or ulceration as a result of undetected entropion. This disease has important welfare aspects if neglected.

• Microphthalmia – vitamin A deficiency, genetic defect in Texels.
• Check for upper eyelid defect ('split eyelid') associated with four horn gene – seen in rare breed units (Hebridean, Manx Loghtan and Jacob breeds).

Check for infectious or traumatic causes.

• Check for parturient trauma – head swollen with oedema of eyelids, use of fingers or eye hooks for delivery.
• If cataract is present, check for border disease.
• Check for infectious disease, e.g. neonatal septicaemia, joint ill, scouring, which can be followed by uveitis.

Note: The clinician may be presented with a patient at a later stage of what is in reality a neonatal condition. Where the diagnosis and treatment have been delayed, the effects may persist due to permanent corneal damage.

Growing lambs and adults

Large numbers or whole group affected, primary lesion is keratoconjunctivitis

• Check for infectious keratoconjunctivitis.

Caused by *Mycoplasma conjunctivae*, *Chlamydia psittaci*.

Other organisms have been isolated from the eyes of sheep but their pathogenicity is not known. These include: *M. arginini*,

M. ovipneumoniae, Acholeplasma oculi, Branhamella ovis, Moraxella bovis, Listeria monocytogenes.

Identification of the causal organism in any particular outbreak is often difficult for several reasons:

(1) Both *Mycoplasma* and *Chlamydia* require the use of special transport media – consult the laboratory for advice.
(2) Mycoplasmas can often be isolated from sheep with healthy eyes.
(3) Isolation of *Chlamydia* requires a deep scraping of conjunctiva with a swab in order to obtain infected cells.
(4) Sampling from eyes which are apparently failing to respond to treatment is usually of little value because of residual effects of antibiotic.

M. conjunctivae is the organism that has been most frequently isolated in outbreaks in the UK in contrast to some countries where *C. psittaci* assumes a greater importance. The true incidence of the two organisms has been difficult to determine because of the problems with isolation and culture. However, diagnosis should include an attempt to identify the cause, as both the course of disease and response to treatment may vary.

Clinical disease often follows the introduction of new animals into a flock, but can exist as persistent infection within a flock due to the presence of carrier animals and variations in immune response. Young animals are generally less severely affected than older ones.

Clinically, an impression *may* be gained that there are two distinct patterns of disease:

C. psittaci
    bilateral involvement
    lymphoid follicles in conjunctival sac
    swelling of conjunctiva
    severe corneal opacity
    poor response to topical treatment
    relapses common.
M. conjunctivae
    may be unilateral
    later development of lymphoid follicles
    corneal opacity less severe
    good response to topical treatment.

It must be emphasized, however, that similar lesions can be produced by both organisms experimentally, and none of the above signs are pathognomonic.

Stages in progression of keratoconjunctivitis
Grade 1 – scleral congestion, excess lachrymation, blepharo-
          spasm.
Grade 2 – corneal inflammation, vascularization, opacity (pan-
          nus) at dorsal aspect.
Grade 3 – corneal ulceration.

Note: *C. psittaci* as an eye infection is not a threat as a source of
abortion, but may give a serological response.

Individual animal affected, excess lachrymation, photophobia, often with corneal involvement

- Check for recent introduction of infectious keratoconjunctivitis, as above. Will spread rapidly to others.
- Check for foreign body in eye, particularly if housed. Foreign
  bodies may be difficult to identify as they rapidly become
  incorporated into the surface of the cornea by the inflammatory reaction.
- Check height of hay racks – these may act as a source of hay
  seeds or dust.
- Check for self mutilation, e.g. following photosensitization or
  facial eczema.

Individual or small numbers affected, no eye lesions, other neurological signs present

- Check for gid or other space-occupying lesion in brain.
- Check for CCN.
- If in late pregnancy, check for pregnancy toxaemia.

Note: Secondary eye damage as a result of prolonged recumbency may occur in such animals. Excess lachrymation and
conjunctivitis may be seen in the early stages of an outbreak of
listeriosis. See chapter 15 for more details.

Individual or small numbers affected, gradual onset of bilateral blindness, no corneal involvement, sheep have access to bracken

- Check for bright blindness (progressive retinal atrophy).

This bilateral condition, caused by prolonged intake of toxic
substances within bracken, rarely affects sheep under 2 years of
age. Affected sheep show a high head carriage and high
stepping gait. The eyes shine in poor light due to excessive

reflection from the retina, and the pupils react poorly to light. Examination with an ophthalmoscope shows narrowing of the blood vessels on the retina, with no inflammatory reaction or opacity in the eye.

Part of flock shows excess lachrymation, no eye lesions, ill-thrift in ewes and lambs

- Check for cobalt deficiency – see chapter 9.

17 Anaemia

Haemorrhagic
  Trauma
  Parasitic
Haemolytic
  Toxins
  Infection
Hypoproliferative
  Nutritional
  Parasitic
  Immunological
Investigation of anaemia
  Young lambs
  Growing lambs
  Adults

With certain exceptions such as overt haemorrhage, anaemia in sheep is a sign of an underlying disease process rather than a primary condition. It follows that evidence of anaemia will be detected during a clinical examination for some other reason, or the finding of anaemia will alert the clinician to search for other signs of disease.

The first indications will usually be pallor of the conjunctivae, third eyelid, mouth and vaginal mucous membranes. This will to some extent be subjective, and dependent upon comparison with contemporaries or other groups of animals.

Mild anaemia is often not noticed unless the animal is examined closely. If the anaemia develops slowly, a fall to below 50% of normal blood parameters can occur without noticeable effect on the animal unless it is exerted, when changes in exercise tolerance, with increased heart and respiratory rates, may be apparent (although these are difficult to interpret anyway as mentioned in the introductory chapter).

Confirmation of anaemia must be by haematological examination, with the finding of lower than normal values for red blood cells, haemoglobin concentration and packed cell volume.

There are three distinct mechanisms by which anaemia may arise: (1) haemorrhagic, (2) haemolytic, (3) depression/hypoproliferative.

Haemorrhagic

Acute
  Obstetric trauma (to ewe)
  Obstetric trauma (to lamb)
  Other trauma
  Umbilical bleeding
Acute/chronic
  Coccidiosis
  Haemonchosis
Chronic
  External parasites
  Chronic fluke

Haemolytic

Copper poisoning
Rape/kale poisoning
Nitrate poisoning
Bacillary haemoglobinuria (*Cl. novyi* type D)

Cl. perfringens type A
Leptospirosis
Haemolytic anaemia may be accompanied by haematuria and followed by jaundice (see chapter 18).

Depression/hypoproliferative

Cobalt deficiency
Copper deficiency
Chronic liver fluke
Chronic parasitic gastroenteritis
Cow colostrum induced anaemia (this is a combination of extravascular haemolysis and bone marrow depression)

Note: Iron deficiency does not occur in adult sheep, and although young lambs housed on a milk diet have been shown to have lower red cell parameters than lambs supplemented with iron, there was no significant effect on growth rates.

Classification of anaemia on morphological appearance of erythrocytes

Although this is done routinely in the investigation of anaemia in man and small animals, it is rarely applied to sheep, but may be of help where a diagnosis is not obvious.

Shape	Hb content	Comment
Normocytic	Normochromic	Normal appearance, chronic PGE Cobalt deficiency
Normocytic	Hypochromic	Chronic blood loss, e.g. haemonchosis
Macrocytic	Normochromic	Cobalt deficiency
Macrocytic	Hypochromic	Recovery after blood loss Subacute/chronic fluke
Microcytic	Normochromic	–
Microcytic	Hypochromic	Chronic blood loss Copper deficiency

Investigation of anaemia (Table 17.1)

Unless the source of blood loss is obvious, a search must be made for the underlying disease process. Except with trauma, most cases will affect a significant number of animals, and may

Table 17.1 Investigation of anaemia

Age group	Haematology (EDTA sample)	Biochemistry (serum or heparinized)	Faeces	PME samples
Lambs <3 weeks	PCV [Coombs test]			Pale carcase Watery blood Pale bone marrow } In cow colostrum anaemia
Lambs <8 weeks	PCV		Coccidial oocysts	Intestinal smear Histology [Liver lesions with T. hydatigena]
Growing lambs	PCV	Co (vitamin B_{12}) Cu	Nematode eggs	Liver (Cu, Co) Worm counts esp. Haemonchus (abomasum, small intestine)
Adults	PCV Ex. for haemolysis	GGT (chronic liver damage) AST ⎱ Acute GLDH ⎰ liver SDH ⎰ damage	Fluke eggs Nematode eggs (Haemonchus)	Liver (fluke) Abomasum Liver, kidney (Cu)

AST = aspartate aminotransferase
GGT = gamma glutamyl transferase
GLDH = glutamate dehydrogenase
PCV = packed cell volume
SDH = sorbitol dehydrogenase

come to light as a result of investigation into poor growth rates or adult weight loss. Aspects of the history which will be relevant include age and number of affected animals, type of pasture, recent pasture improvements, concentrate feeding (especially cattle or pig food), access to cattle minerals, parasite control measures. It may be helpful to sacrifice an affected animal and carry out a full postmortem examination if the cause is not obvious.

Sample taking

Where a group of animals is involved, at least six samples should be taken for any haematological, biochemical or parasitological examination.

For haematological examination, EDTA (ethylenediamine-tetra-acetic acid) is the anticoagulant of choice. Heparin and OxF can be used for red cell counts but are not suitable for WBC counts.

Cobalt (B_{12}) and copper estimation require a serum or heparinized blood sample.

Normal range of red cell values

RBC 5–12 × 10^{12}/l
Hb 8–15 g/dl
PCV 0.24–0.40
Reticulocytes 0%
MCV 25–40 fl
MCHC 31–36%

The commonest causes of anaemia according to age group are given below.

Young lambs (<4 weeks)

- Haemorrhage – external, e.g. from umbilical vessel, internal, e.g. liver rupture or other obstetric trauma.
- Cow colostrum-induced anaemia. A history of feeding cow colostrum within the first 24 h, with anaemia developing at 6–14 days is virtually diagnostic. Packed cell volume (PCV) is useful and rapid to screen others exposed. PCV <0.20 is significant, although clinical illness may not be seen until <0.12. Can be confirmed by direct Coombs test which shows presence of bovine IgG on erythrocytes in most cases. PM shows pale carcase with small amount of watery blood, pale creamy bone marrow.
- Migrating *Taenia hydatigena* larvae in liver may cause acute haemorrhage. Occasionally seen in orphan lambs reared in close proximity to farm dogs.

Growing lambs

- Check for cobalt deficiency (blood biochemistry)
- Check for copper deficiency (blood biochemistry)
- Check for *Haemonchus* infection (no scouring, bottle jaw) – faeces sample for nematode eggs, but species cannot be differentiated.
- Check for PGE (concurrent scouring) faeces sample as above.
- Check for coccidiosis (blood in faeces, may occur *before* oocyst production). May require PME to confirm.
- Check for acute fluke – recent grazing history, serum or

plasma sample for liver enzymes. Aspartate aminotransferase (AST), glutamate dehydrogenase (GLDH) and sorbitol dehydrogenase (SDH) indicate acute liver damage. PME to confirm.

Adults

- Check for acute/chronic fluke.
- Check for *Haemonchus* infection.
- Check for copper poisoning (anaemia followed by jaundice if survive).
- Check for rape/kale poisoning (less susceptible than cattle).
- Check for lice infestation (should be rare because of dipping campaign).
- Check for nitrate poisoning – nitrate is non-toxic but is converted to nitrite in rumen. This is absorbed and produces methaemoglobinaemia (chocolate brown blood), with methaemoglobinuria.

18 Jaundice

Prehepatic
  Toxins
  Infections
Hepatic
  Toxins
  Infections
Posthepatic
  Obstructive
Investigation

As with anaemia, jaundice is a sign of a disease process, and not a primary condition itself. It will be vital evidence of a pathological condition such as a haemolytic crisis or liver dysfunction, and will be identified during clinical or postmortem examination.

Jaundice arises from an increase in the bilirubin content of the blood giving rise clinically to yellow pigmentation of the mucous membranes and sclera (see Figure 18.1). At PME there is yellowing of all the body tissues, particularly the liver.

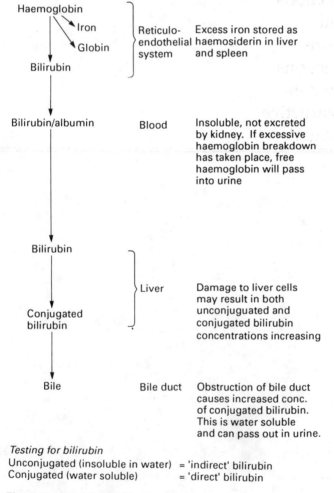

Testing for bilirubin
Unconjugated (insoluble in water)   = 'indirect' bilirubin
Conjugated (water soluble)   = 'direct' bilirubin

Figure 18.1 Breakdown of haemoglobin

Note: Some sheep possess a natural yellow pigmentation of the body fat, and this should not be mistaken for jaundice – check the mucous membranes to differentiate.

Jaundice usually is caused by one of three factors.

An excess breakdown of erythrocytes by haemolysis (prehepatic jaundice)

There is no impairment to bile flow, and it is the unconjugated (indirect) bilirubin content of the blood which is raised.

Causes

- Copper poisoning
- Kale poisoning
- Onion poisoning
- *Cl. perfringens* type A
- *Cl. novyi* type D
- *Leptospira pomona.*

See also chapter 17 on haemolytic anaemia.

Liver dysfunction

In this type, the conjugated (direct) and unconjugated (indirect) bilirubin content of the blood are raised, because of inability of damaged liver cells to conjugate, and interference with bile excretion.

Causes

- Photosensitization, (chronic fluke), infections of the liver

Bile duct obstruction (posthepatic jaundice)

In this type the conjugated (direct) bilirubin content of the blood is raised because of back-pressure from blocked bile duct.

Causes

- (Chronic fluke), tumours, other obstructive conditions

Investigation of jaundice

Important aspects of history taking include the following:

- Incidence (single case or many affected)

- Age
- Feeding/grazing
- Concentrate feeding
- Access to minerals
- Parasite status
- Local knowledge of poisonous plants.

Note: Sheep with copper poisoning may be found dead, and it is important that all contacts should be thoroughly examined. Severe anaemia may be present in the early stage of the disease before the onset of jaundice.

Blood sampling

(1) EDTA sample for haematology and bilirubin concentrations. Normal values for bilirubin:
Total <10.0 μmol/l
Direct< 1.7 μmol/l
(2) Serum or plasma (heparinized) sample is very helpful. The most useful tests are:
Acute liver disease – AST, GLDH, SDH
Chronic liver disease – gamma glutamyl transferase (GGT)
Total protein and albumin content
Phylloerythrin content (in acute phase only)

Note: SDH is an accurate indicator of acute liver damage, but must be assayed within 4 h of sampling.
(3) Heparinized blood or serum for copper estimation.

Postmortem material

Liver and kidney (100 g) for copper content.
    The most common causes of jaundice can be linked to particular age groups.

Young lambs

- Check for cow colostrum feeding.

Note: Although there is excessive red cell destruction, jaundice is not usually a feature of this condition.

- Check for possibility of leptospirosis.

Growing and adult sheep

- Check for copper poisoning. PME if deaths occur, blood Cu in contacts, liver enzymes AST, GLDH, SDH. Check for source of excess copper – cattle concentrates, cattle minerals, grass spread with pig slurry.

There is considerable breed and strain variation in sensitivity to copper in the diet. Diets which cause toxicity in some breeds may lead to swayback lambs in others, e.g. the Texel is very susceptible to copper poisoning, the Scottish Blackface may produce swayback lambs on a similar diet. An extreme example of susceptibility to copper poisoning is the North Ronaldsay breed, which has developed a highly efficient system for obtaining copper from its normal diet of seaweed, and is extremely difficult to keep alive on a conventional diet.

Supplementation with copper, therefore, should only be carried out where a known problem exists, or after sampling a representative number of animals. The most important influence on copper uptake is the amount of molybdenum in the diet. In winter, sheep grazing bare fields ingest considerable amounts of soil which increases molybdenum intake. If there is prolonged snow cover, the soil intake is reduced, therefore more copper is absorbed. In cases where flocks previously outwintered are housed, particular care needs to be taken over copper supplementation, since copper absorption from the diet increases in two ways – because soil ingestion does not take place, and from the natural copper content of concentrate feeds.

- Check for rape/kale feeding.
- Check for severe fluke.

Note: Jaundice is rarely a feature of chronic fluke even in presence of high fluke numbers and severe liver damage.

- Check for recent drug administration.
- Check for photosensitization – oedema and irritation of head and ears, followed by drying and crusting of skin. See also chapter 20 on skin lesions.

Photosensitization arises in three ways:

(1) plant poisoning, e.g. St Johns Wort,
(2) aberrant pigment synthesis (not recognized in sheep in UK),
(3) hepatogenous – liver damage, caused by plant toxins, fungal toxins or drugs, interfering with excretion of phylloerythrin which is a normal product of ruminant digestion. Jaundice is not always a feature.

- Other rare causes of jaundice such as tumours are likely to be found at PME only.

19 Abdominal distension/abdominal pain

Acute distension
  Obstructive
  Abdominal catastrophe
  Motility dysfunction
Chronic distension
  Pregnancy-associated problems
  Nutritional
  Gastrointestinal dysfunction
  Cardiac/liver dysfunction
Pain
  Acute gastrointestinal obstruction
  Parasitism
  Parturition-associated
  Urinary obstruction

Although abdominal distension and abdominal pain can and frequently do exist as separate clinical entities, they may be linked in aetiology. Factors which cause distension may also cause pain, or pain may result from the distension.

There is one important cause of abdominal distension which the client may not recognize as abnormal, namely extreme fetal overload, which may nevertheless place maternal survival in jeopardy. The manipulation of nutrition to maximize reproductive potential, or the use of artificial means to increase litter size, in conjunction with unchanged dependence upon a ruminant digestive system, have produced a situation in some animals where late pregnancy *is* a disease!

Diagnosis will be made easier by consideration of the sex, age and reproductive status of the patient. In addition, the speed of onset in the case of abdominal distension will be of great significance.

Abdominal distension (Figure 19.1)

At birth

If the lamb is delivered with a distended abdomen

- Check incidence, breed, cross – possible genetic origin.
- Check for other abnormalities – achondroplasia, kidney abnormality.
- Check for other evidence of abortion or stillbirths – premature lambs often give the appearance of a distended or 'watery' belly.

Neonate

If rapid onset:

- Check for high alimentary obstruction : pyloric stenosis, pyloric obstruction (milk curd), gastric torsion.
- Check for watery mouth – excess salivation, depression, loss of appetite (this will be a flock problem).
- Check castration technique – urethral occlusion.

If slow onset:

- Check for low alimentary obstruction, imperforate anus, or other congenital alimentary defect.
- Check for ascites (paracentesis) – congenital heart defect or kidney defect.

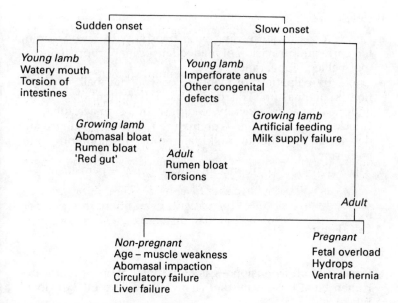

Figure 19.1 Abdominal distension

Growing lambs

If rapid onset:

- Check for abomasal bloat – almost invariably in artificially milk-fed lambs on infrequent large feeds. These will either be 'pets' or in multiple units fed on milk substitutes with concentrates available. Access to grass as well appears to be an aggravating factor.
- Check for 'red gut' (torsion of intestines). This is an abdominal catastrophe, and the lamb is likely to be found dead. If seen alive, there is severe abdominal distension and pain with rapid deterioration and death within a short time. This condition is thought to be caused by rapid throughput of highly digestible food, with excess gas production in the intestines. Instability develops, followed by torsion of the intestines and occlusion of the anterior mesenteric artery.
- Check for true rumen bloat (pass stomach tube). This may be due to sudden change of diet, low fibre intake, high clover content.

If slow onset:

- Check for artificial feeding with poor growth rate, weaning too early and provision of inadequate or inappropriate food – 'pot-bellied' appearance.
- Check by palpation for evidence of wool/hair ball, or excess fibre in abomasum. This may cause intermittent obstruction, and may be aggravated by feeding with a stomach tube.
- Check for 'grass scours' – premature rumen dependence and development, due to milk failure or mismothering after gathering.
- Check for concurrent anaemia and debility – parasitism.

Adult (Figure 19.2)

If rapid onset:

- Check site of distension – gas high in left abdomen indicates rumen bloat caused by diet change, low fibre intake, clover intake.
- Check for abdominal catastrophe, intestinal torsion. Rapid pulse, rapid deterioration, death.

If slow onset:

- Check stage of pregnancy – fetal overload, poor body condition, fetuses palpable.
- Check age and reproductive history – muscle stretch after multiple pregnancies.
- Check for hydrops amnii/allantois – bilateral distension, fetuses not palpable, may be fluid wave detectable. Scanning may be helpful.
- Check for abdominal wall trauma – ventral hernia.
- Check food quality – low digestibility of fibre may cause excess rumen fill.
- Check for abomasal impaction – palpable in low right abdomen. Results from inadequate rumination (molar tooth disease), or part of 'vagal indigestion' syndrome.
- Check heart – circulatory failure may give ascites (do paracentesis, avoiding rumen area).
- Check for dependent oedema – chronic fluke, mastitis, debility.

Other causes such as neoplasms are unlikely to be diagnosed until PME.

171

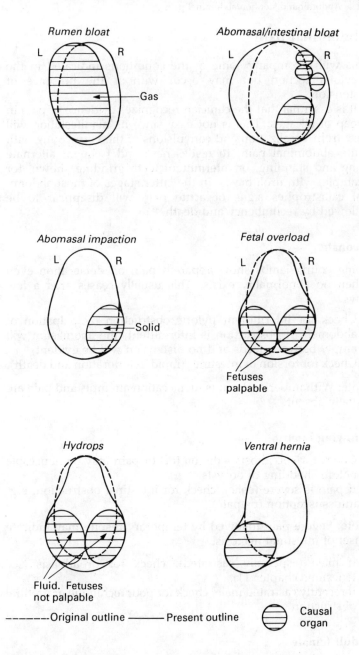

Figure 19.2 Shape of abdomen in cross-section as aid to diagnosis

Abdominal pain

This will accompany some of the conditions indicated in the previous section but may occur without the presence of distension.

It is essential that the clinician recognizes evidence of pain in sheep of all ages. This is not easy since its manifestation will vary from vocalization and convulsions of the very young with acute abdominal pain, to restlessness and frequent alternate lying and standing, or intermittent teeth grinding shown, for example, with urolithiasis. In the latter stages of most abdominal catastrophes signs of acute pain will disappear to be followed by recumbency and death.

Neonate

Some young lambs show apparent pain on defaecation even when no abnormality exists. This usually ceases after a few days.

- Check for intermittent pyloric obstruction by palpation of abdomen. If obstruction is intermittent, the abomasum will empty between feeds and no distension will be evident.
- Check for torsion of intestines (rapid deterioration and death).

Note: With imperforate anus, defaecation attempts and pain are usually absent.

Growing lamb

- Check for coccidiosis – discomfort or pain may be noticeable before shedding of oocysts.
- If pain is severe (colic), check for intestinal obstruction, e.g. intussusception (palpate).

Note: Severe pain followed by temporary respite may indicate onset of intestinal necrosis.

- If male (especially castrated), check for urolithiasis (see tenesmus chapter 11).
- If recently castrated male, check for poor technique or urethral obstruction.

Adult female

- Check for evidence of abortion or parturition.

- Check for torsion of uterus if parturition appears imminent but no progress (vaginal examination may show characteristic twists, but torsion anterior to cervix may not be detectable).
- Check for postparturient infection/trauma.

Adult male

- Check for urinary obstruction.
- Check for inguinal herniation.
- Check for traumatic balanitis.

20 Wool loss/skin lesions

Lambs
  Fleece abnormalities
  Infections
Growing lambs and adults
  Non-pruritic lesions on hairy areas
  Pruritic lesions on hairy areas
  Wool loss without pruritis
  Wool loss with pruritis

The clinician must keep in mind that hair and wool are products of actively growing cells, even though the visible external structures are 'biologically' dead. Any nutritional deprivation, systemic disease, or stress affecting the function of the body as a whole is likely to have a direct effect on these structures, particularly on wool production, though there may be a time lag in the appearance of such changes. Severe illness or debility will soon lead to weakening of the wool fibres or to shedding of the fleece, which is hastened by using the wool to catch or restrain the animal. In other animals suffering more chronic illness or undernutrition, the effects may appear as thinning of the fibres, which can be seen macroscopically or can be detected by applying tension to the staple which will break at any weak point. This weakness is referred to as 'tenderness'. Normal healthy wool has a very high tensile strength.

In addition to this loss of wool as a result of acute or chronic illness, it should be recognized that seasonal partial or complete loss occurs in some breeds. For example, primitive sheep such as the Soay shed or moult the fleece, and some longwool breeds and crosses, particularly older animals, may lose wool along the spine in the late spring. Wool can also be mechanically removed by young lambs which often jump on to the backs of the ewes when playing.

These types of wool loss or poor growth are additional to and separate from the specific skin diseases which may themselves cause wool loss by affecting the follicles, or as a result of self-inflicted damage because of pruritis.

The vast majority of cases of skin lesions or wool loss will be seen in grazing lambs or adult sheep, and will be secondary to nutritional, infectious or parasitic disease, but there are a small number of conditions which will be apparent at or soon after birth.

Neonatal and very young lambs

Poor or underdeveloped fleece

This is a sign of prematurity.

● Check for infectious causes of abortion if several lambs are affected.

Abnormally hairy and/or pigmented fleece

● Check for border disease. Affected lambs show abnormal

number of 'halo hairs' (long kempy fibres), often in conjunction with neurological signs ('hairy shakers'). Such lambs are virus positive, and were exposed to infection *in utero* before about day 85 of gestation. Abnormal brown or black pigmentation in normally unpigmented breeds may also indicate the presence of border disease.

Note: Normal lambs from Welsh ewes or crosses often show some pigmentation which fades with increasing age. The birth coat may also show marked variations, with patches of hairy and non-hairy coat on the same animal. Border disease should not be diagnosed in such animals without further supporting evidence, e.g. neurological signs, positive serology, virus isolation.

Proliferative lesions on lips and/or inside mouth

- Check for orf – this is particularly common in groups of artificially reared lambs, and can appear within a few days of birth. Check teat hygiene, although if lambs are being fed with a multi-teat unit it is almost impossible to prevent spread through the whole group. If lambs are sucking the ewe, check for teat lesions. Take care in handling – orf is a zoonosis.

Loss of hair and horn, recumbency

- Check for 'redfoot'. This hereditary condition affects Scottish Blackface sheep and their crosses, and is seen within the first few weeks of life. It is progressive, with ulceration of oral mucous membranes and cornea, with death resulting from infection or starvation.

Loss of wool, no systemic illness

- This may occasionally result from an allergy to artificial milk, or possibly, rarely, to the ewe's milk.

Grazing lambs and adults

Although the client is likely to call for help on the basis of 'wool loss' or 'skin lesions', this will usually be accompanied by complaints of 'scratching' or 'itching', or comment that these features are absent. The number of animals affected will also be

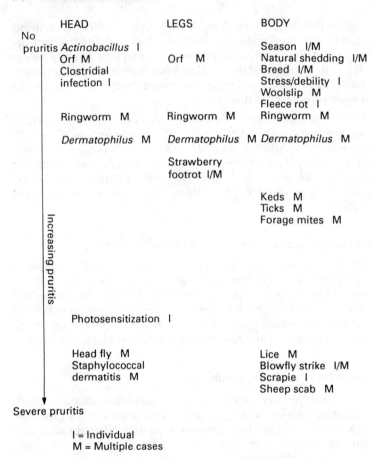

Figure 20.1 Site and degree of pruritis as aid to diagnosis

significant. The delineation into these groups may not always be clear cut, however, and no diagnosis should be excluded on the presence or absence of pruritis alone (see Figure 20.1).

Individual animals, non-woolled areas affected

If the client is observant, the first case of an infectious condition may be noticed. Alternatively, some conditions of low pathogenicity may be confined to a single case.

Lesions generally non-pruritic

- Face swelling with abscess formation – check for actinobacillosis – multiple fibrosed nodules, some of which may discharge pus, are present in the subcutaneous tissue, often forming a chain along the course of the lymphatics.
- Pustules in hair follicles on lips, muzzle or perineum of lambs, or on the udder of lactating ewes – check for staphylococcal folliculitis. Scabs may form, but these are insignificant compared with lesions of orf or staphylococcal dermatitis. The conditions can be differentiated on the grounds of severity, but dry scabs and swabs of lesions can be submitted for viral and bacteriological investigation if necessary.
- Strawberry-like lesions on face or legs – check for orf virus. These usually affect only individual animals within a group, and may indicate an inability to respond effectively to the virus. See below.
- Persistent lesions of hyperkeratosis on poll (especially of rams) or ears – check for persistent orf infection – see below.
- Swelling and oedema of head, fever and rapid death. Check for clostridial infection of wounds, e.g. rams fighting. Check vaccination history.

Lesions generally pruritic

- Check for photosensitization – face swelling followed by exudation and crusting of unpigmented skin especially head, ears, legs and perineal area. Some of affected skin may slough off, especially the ear tips. Jaundice occurs in some cases.

Photosensitization occurs because of the presence within the body of photodynamic substances which may arise in two different ways in the UK:

(1) Ingestion of plants containing a photodynamic substance, e.g. St John's wort, or treatment with certain drugs such as phenothiazine.
(2) Hepatogenous, i.e. as a result of liver damage caused by plants containing toxins, e.g. rape, fungal toxins, or certain drugs. Bog asphodel has been associated with photosensitization, but it is now thought that this arises from fungal toxins on the plants, rather than from the plant itself. In all these cases there is a build-up of photodynamic phylloerythrin, a breakdown product of chlorophyll, which is normally metabolized in the liver.

Many animals, non-woolled areas affected

The conditions described above may appear in more than one animal, but where a number of animals are affected, the cause is likely to be infectious. Diagnosis will be assisted by sampling typical lesions by taking scab material, swabs from beneath scabs, and scrapings from active areas of lesions as necessary. Table 20.1 lists aids to diagnosis.

Table 20.1 Diagnostic aids for wool loss/skin lesions

	Gross Pathology	Site	Microbiology	Parasitology
Staphylococcal dermatitis	Deep ulceration Black scabs	Face	Haemolytic staphylococcus	
Ringworm	Dry, crusted scabs	Head, body if shorn		Fungal spores
Mycotic dermatitis (*Dermatophilus*)	Exudation, matted wool, raised scabs, superficial raw areas under scabs	Body, face, ears	Gram +ve filamentous cocci	
Wool rot	Confined to wool fibres – coloration	Body especially back	*Pseudomonas aeruginosa*	
Orf	Vesicles, scabs, proliferative lesions	Mouth, lips, legs, teats, prepuce	Virus (with electron microscope)	
Sheep scab	Exudation, yellow crusts, intense pruritis, marked wool loss	Body		*Psoroptes* *notifiable
Scrapie	Self-inflicted lesions, neurological signs	Body, tailhead	–	–
Photo-sensitization	Exudation, crusting, skin loss	Head, ears, legs back	–	–
Debility	No skin lesions weak wool fibres	Body random	–	–
Wool slip	No skin lesions recently shorn	Body: back, flanks	– –	(occasionally forage mites)
Other external parasites	Parasites visible	Depends on species involved	–	Lice keds ticks blowfly larvae

Lesions generally non-pruritic

- Scabs on mouth and lips (in very early stages papules and vesicles present) – check for orf (contagious pustular dermatitis). This common infection caused by a parapox virus may also be found on the teats of lactating ewes, inside the mouth of young lambs and on the genitalia of rams. In some individual animals, the virus may persist causing proliferative lesions on the head and legs (see above). Diagnosis is confirmed by submitting scabs for demonstration of the virus with an electron microscope. *Care should be taken in handling material since orf is a zoonosis.*
- Raised crusts which separate or can be lifted off leaving raw areas beneath – check for mycotic dermatitis (caused by the bacterium *Dermatophilus congolensis*). This may affect the face and ears particularly in lambs, and the scrotum of rams. Make impression smears of the underside of freshly removed scabs and stain with Gram's stain. Shows Gram-positive branching filaments breaking into multiple rows of Gram-positive cocci. If further confirmation is required, submit samples to laboratory for FAT (fluorescent antibody test) or isolation. The same organism infects woolled areas of older sheep causing 'lumpy wool', and in combination with orf virus, causes strawberry footrot in lambs. See below.
- Proliferative scabby lesions which bleed when scabs are removed affecting coronary and lower leg areas – check for strawberry footrot. This is generally considered to be caused by a combination of orf and *Dermatophilus* infection.
- Multiple dry crusted areas on head and/or legs – check for ringworm (usually *Trichophyton verrucosum*). Take skin scrapings and hairs from edge of lesion, mix with potassium hydroxide and examine for spores. There will usually be contact with calves or buildings in which calves have been reared. *Ringworm is a zoonosis.*
- Lesions affecting the prepuce of rams or the vulva of ewes – although mycoplasmas and ureaplasms have been isolated their significance is not known. There appears to be no effect on fertility.
- Lesions affecting interdigital space, with lameness – check for scald (see chapter 14). Remember the possibility of foot and mouth disease!

Lesions pruritic (Figure 20.2)

Some of the conditions described above may become pruritic, particularly if secondary infection takes place, or during the

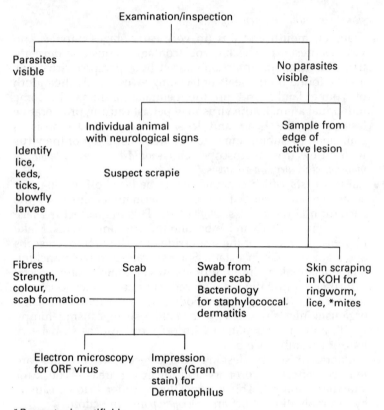

Psoroptes is notifiable

Figure 20.2 Stages in diagnosis of pruritic skin lesions and wool loss

healing process, therefore should not be excluded on presence or absence of pruritis alone. In addition there are two important causes of pruritic lesions affecting usually the heads of many animals.

● If wounds around base of horns in summer, suspect head fly (*Hydrotea irritans*). Affects mainly young horned sheep, but may also affect other sheep with skin damage on the head, e.g. rams fighting. When flies are active in still warm weather, affected animals can be seen shaking their heads and trying to avoid the swarms of insects. Sheep with wool cover on the head are less likely to be affected.

- If severe ulcerated lesions are present around the eyes, nose, ears and horns, particularly if animals are being trough fed, suspect staphylococcal dermatitis. Ulcers bleed easily, become covered with black scabs and hair is lost from the surrounding area. The severe clinical picture should suggest a diagnosis, but this can be confirmed by isolation of haemolytic *Staph. aureus* from the lesions.

Individual animals, woolled areas affected

No pruritis present, no skin lesions

- If loss is zonal around neck or along spine, check for natural shedding or delayed shearing. Masham and mule sheep often lose wool prematurely from these areas. As previously mentioned, some primitive sheep shed the fleece naturally in early summer.
- If loss is random, check for acute or chronic illness, undernutrition, debility or other stress.
- If sheep are winter shorn, suspect 'wool slip' – new wool growth is lost particularly from the spine and flank areas. This condition is thought to be caused by excess cortisol production as a result of a combination of stress factors associated with housing and shearing, but occasionally may be caused by feed mites, in which case some pruritis would be expected.

Pruritis present (see Figure 20.2)

- If in summer months, check for blowfly strike. Affected animals are restless, show excessive tail twitching and foot stamping, frequently turning the head to attempt to nibble the lesion. The most commonly affected area is soiled wool around the tail, but other parts of the body and even the feet may be involved. Lesions, which are intensely pruritic, may be difficult to locate in the early stages simply appearing as areas of damp wool, but a characteristic smell soon develops and maggots should be found on careful searching.
- If 'nibbling' reflex is present in absence of ectoparasites, check for scrapie. Can be seen in sheep as young as 2 years (recently in even younger animals), although most cases are in older animals. Self-inflicted skin lesions may be present, as well as neurological signs such as incoordination, hyperexcitability (see chapter 15). There is no confirmatory test in live animals, final diagnosis depending on characteristic brain histology.

Many animals, woolled areas affected

No pruritis, no skin lesions

Those conditions listed as affecting individual animals may also affect more than one of a group, i.e.

- natural shedding – breed
- undernutrition on flock basis, particularly in late pregnancy, e.g. cases of pregnancy toxaemia
- woolslip if winter shorn

In addition

- If wool growth generally is poor in quality and/or quantity, check for micronutrient deficiency. Copper and cobalt deficiency both have effects on fleece growth as well as leading to ill thrift.
- Check for other chronic disease such as coccidiosis, parasitic gastroenteritis. See chapter 9.

Skin lesions or abnormal wool present, little pruritis

- Check for mycotic dermatitis (lumpy wool). *D. congolensis* commonly affects fleeced areas as well as hairy areas as described above. Lesions most commonly appear on the back, and consist of an exudative dermatitis, the exudate drying causing the wool to mat with scab formation. In early cases this may only be seen when the fleece is parted, but becomes more obvious as the disease progresses. Diagnosis is confirmed by staining impression smears of scabs. See above. In some cases pruritis is present.
- Check for ringworm – this is rare on woolled areas, but may occur in sheep exposed to infection soon after shearing, e.g. in winter housing with calf contact. Confirm with examination of hairs and skin scrapings from active part of lesion (zoonosis).
- If matting of the wool with abnormal pigmentation, usually yellow or greenish-blue is present, suspect fleece rot (canary stain). This is thought to be caused by pigment-producing bacteria such as *Pseudomonas aeruginosa*, particularly in prolonged wet weather. Affected fleeces are downgraded.

Note: Yellow pigmentation of grease which easily washes out is commonly found in some breeds, particularly longwools.

Pruritis present (see Figure 20.2)

Most conditions with pruritis will involve skin lesions; if not a part of the primary cause, they will become apparent as a result of self-mutilation. Some skin lesions which are not initially pruritic may become so during the healing process or as a result of secondary infection.

There are a few transitory conditions where pruritis occurs without the development of skin lesions, but may give an inexperienced owner cause for concern:

- In hot weather immediately pre-shearing, sheep in heavy fleeces may rub against fences, hedges, etc.
- In warm humid weather, small flies and midges cause irritation, with sheep showing sudden head shaking, foot stamping, and alternate lying and standing. This behaviour can be seen in housed sheep as well as in those at grass.
- Store lambs on *ad libitum* complete diet may show sporadic attacks of pruritis, possibly due to transient food allergy.

As mentioned above, some cases of mycotic dermatitis and ringworm may also show significant pruritis. However, the majority of incidents involving many animals with severe pruritis will be parasitic in origin.

- Check for sheep scab (*Psoroptes communis var. ovis*). Affected sheep show intense irritation with exudate drying to form yellow crusts in the fleece which become moist and matted. Areas of wool are soon lost because of continuous rubbing. *This is a notifiable disease. Consult Divisional Veterinary Officer if suspected.*
- Check for fly strike – this can affect more than one animal if weather conditions are favourable for fly activity, particularly if dagging has been neglected.
- If pruritis is less severe, check for lice, keds, ticks or mites.

Damalinia ovis is a biting louse and is found mostly around the neck and back areas. It has a rounded head.

Linognathus ovillus is a sucking louse and is found mainly around the head. It is blue in colour with a conical head.

Melophagus ovinus (ked) is much larger than lice and is readily visible, unlike lice which may require careful examination to spot.

Tyroglyphus (forage mite) occasionally caused problems in housed sheep and requires skin brushings to identify.

Ixodes ricinus (castor bean ticks) are found mainly on the hairy areas of the head, neck, axilla and groin in spring and autumn. If these are found, consider the possibility of tick-borne diseases as well as tick worry.

Haemaphysalis punctata (festooned tick) is occasionally found in southern Britain.

Note: The presence of lice or keds indicates poor dipping practice, since the compulsory double dipping for sheep scab should have eliminated these ectoparasites.

21 Respiratory disease

Lambs
  Trauma
  Expansion failure
  Inhalation
  Infections
Growing lambs
  Acute infections
  Chronic infections
  Parasitism
  Inhalation
Adults
  Acute infections
  Chronic infections
  Upper respiratory obstruction
Postmortem

The standard criteria used in the antemortem diagnosis of respiratory disease in other species are very limited in application to the sheep, yet the two statements 'pneumonia is the single greatest cause of death in the sheep' and 'pasteurellosis is the most over-diagnosed disease of sheep' are both true, and not contradictory as might appear at first glance.

The respiratory rate of normal sheep shows wide variations according to factors such as weather conditions, fleece cover and fatness. It can be very rapid (>100/min), sometimes with open-mouth breathing, in the full fleeced ewe, on a hot day in humid conditions, even at rest. If the sheep is fat and is driven, then the rate may become dangerously high, still in a normal healthy animal. A shorn ewe at rest on a cool day may well have a very low respiratory rate (<20/min).

In advanced pregnancy, when reproductive products may occupy in excess of 60% of abdominal volume, the respiratory rate may also be raised to one which, to the inexperienced observer, would suggest pathological change. Thus, respiratory rate alone, without taking into account other factors, is a very unreliable guide to the presence or absence of disease.

Auscultation of the chest may give some limited information in the young lamb or newly shorn ewe, but restraint for examination may exaggerate the sounds heard. It should also be borne in mind that rumen sounds can normally be heard over a large area of the ribs, posterior to approximately the sixth rib on the left side.

Coughing, nasal discharge and/or fluid escape from the nares are significant. The type of respiration may also be of significance, although it should be remembered that in the normal sheep it is mainly abdominal rather than thoracic in nature.

Body temperature is also of limited significance in the sheep being subject to the same wide variations as respiratory rate.

To complete the limitations of clinical diagnosis, the sheep seems to have a very low innate resistance to respiratory infection, which, combined with the usual infrequency of examination by the owner, means that the animal is often found dead before any clinical examination can be carried out (except in case of chronic or slow viral diseases). It follows that the vast majority of respiratory disease is diagnosed at PME, and it is in the interpretation of postmortem findings that the clinician will be able to apply expertise.

In addition to physical causes such as trauma and inhalation pneumonia, the following organisms are frequently involved in the pathology of respiratory disorders of sheep.

Bacteria

- *Pasteurella haemolytica* (this is also a normal inhabitant of the upper respiratory tract) – biotypes A and T and at least 15 serotypes.
  Biotype A causes both systemic and pneumonic disease.
  Biotype T causes systemic disease mainly in young sheep.
- *Pasteurella multocida.*
- *Actinomyces (Corynebacterium) pyogenes* causes abscesses.
- *Streptococci.*
- Coliforms.

Mycoplasmas

- *Mycoplasma ovipneumoniae* – together with *P. haemolytica* causes atypical pneumonia.
- *M. arginini.*

Viruses

- Retrovirus causes pulmonary adenomatosis.
- Lentivirus causes maedi visna.
- Parainfluenzae 3 (PI3) virus – sometimes as primary disease but mainly as a factor in *Pasteurella* outbreaks (this may also be a normal pathogen of the upper respiratory tract).
- Adenovirus
- Reovirus 1,2 and 3   } significance not clear.
- Respiratory syncytial virus

Parasites

- *Dictyocaulus filaria.*
- *Muellerius capillaris*
- *Protostrongylus rufescens*   } Little or no clinical significance.
- *Cystocaulus ocreatus*

Frequently, there will be coexistence of two or more infective agents, particularly *Pasteurella* with pulmonary adenomatosis, or *Pasteurella* with *Mycoplasmas* in atypical pneumonia.

From this formidable list, a diagnosis can only be made with confidence on a combination of history taking, age of the patient (Table 21.1), postmortem lesions, bacteriology, histology, parasitology and serology where appropriate.

Antemortem diagnosis of respiratory disease

The following points may assist in diagnosis in the live animal, but it must be emphasized that confirmation may require postmortem examination of representative animals.

Neonate

Here, changes in respiratory rate are more often of significance than in the older sheep, but may not necessarily indicate lesions in the lungs or upper respiratory tract. A raised body temperature is also more significant than in the older animal, but it should be remembered that hypothermia will soon intervene if the young lamb ceases to feed for any length of time.

Note: In the neonate, the clinical pattern of respiratory infections is septicaemic rather than pneumonic. Depression and death are likely to occur before thoracic changes progress to the point at which dyspnoea would be apparent.

Dyspnoea/tachypnoea

- Check for trauma of the rib cage – parturient trauma, or treading injury.
- Check for pharyngeal/laryngeal oedema – head only presentation.
- Check for failure of lung expansion – neonatal acute respiratory distress syndrome – prematurity or surfactant failure.
- Check heart for congenital defects.
- Check for inhalation pneumonia – often associated with artificial or force feeding – rattling respiration, milky discharge down nostrils.
- Check for evidence of anaemia – umbilical bleeding, or cow colostrum induced.
- Check for septicaemic pasteurellosis.

Growing lambs

As noted above, the clinical picture of diseases caused by potential thoracic pathogens changes from being primarily septicaemic in the very young, to primarily thoracic in the growing animal.

Table 21.1 Age incidence of common causes of respiratory problems

	Individual	Multiple

Neonate	Trauma (ribs)
	Neonatal respiratory
	  distress
	Postdystocia oedema
	Haemorrhage
	Inhalation (milk)
		Septicaemic pasteurellosis
		Nutritional myopathy
		  (intercostal muscles)
		Cow colostrum anaemia

Growing
  lambs
	Inhalation pneumonia
	  (drench, dip)
		Inhalation
		  (drench, dip)
		Atypical pneumonia
		Acute pasteurellosis
		Chronic pasteurellosis
		Parasitic bronchitis
		Nutritional myopathy

Adults	As above +
	  laryngeal chondritis
		As above +
		  pulmonary adenomatosis
		  maedi

Table 21.2 Speed of onset of respiratory disease

	Acute	Chronic
Neonate	Trauma Neonatal respiratory distress Postdystocia oedema Muscular dystrophy Haemorrhage Inhalation	
Growing lambs	Acute pasteurellosis Inhalation Muscular dystrophy	Chronic pasteurellosis Atypical pneumonia Parasitic bronchitis
Adults	Laryngeal chondritis Acute pasteurellosis	Maedi Pulmonary adenomatosis Chronic pasteurellosis Chronic nasal obstruction

Dyspnoea

- Check by auscultation for evidence of areas of consolidation. These may indicate atypical pneumonia, viral infection or pasteurellosis, or a combination of organisms. Often outbreaks begin with some sudden deaths. PME is required for differentiation. Paired sera may assist with retrospective diagnosis of viral involvement, but are not very helpful with pasteurella because of number of serotypes involved.
- Check for drenching routine – inhalation pneumonia, or stress induced pasteurellosis.

- Check for nutritional myopathy affecting respiratory muscles (blood sample for CK and GSH-Px estimations).

Chronic cough

- Check for atypical pneumonia – postmortem confirmation.
- Check for parasitic bronchitis – faeces samples for larval identification (check type of wormer used – some (cheap) drugs are not effective against lungworms).
- Check for chronic pleurisy, pleural adhesions or effusion.

Nasal discharge

- Check for viral infection and/or pasteurellosis as above. Isolation of *P. haemolytica* from nasal swabs does *not* confirm diagnosis since it is present in most normal sheep. Paired sera with rising titres for viruses such as PI3 may help to indicate viral involvement.
- Check for transient stress-induced upper respiratory infection (non-febrile with little or no systemic involvement).
- If unilateral, may be *Oestrus ovis* infection, although there is no easy method of diagnosis unless parasites are sneezed out.
- Check for excessively dusty conditions.

Any of above plus reduced weight gain or emaciation

- Check by auscultation for chronic lung damage, possible chronic pasteurellosis or neonatal septicaemia with multiple abscesses in lung tissue plus pleurisy.

Older sheep

The clinical picture of a recent infection with pasteurellosis and/ or viral infection will not differ from that shown in growing lambs. When these infections have become long-standing, or where chronic viral infections are involved, chronic weight loss becomes an additional diagnostic feature.

Chronic cough with weight loss

- Check by auscultation for pleurisy and areas of consolidation.
- Check for excessive fluid in airways (wheelbarrow test) – pathognomonic for pulmonary adenomatosis (SPA).
- Check breed or breed contact (imports) in case of maedi (MV) (serological evidence of infection, and a few clinical cases have

been found in some indigenous sheep, presumably originating from contact with imported sheep. Check by serology if necessary).

Note: Slow viral infection will primarily affect adults from 2 to 4 years in the case of pulmonary adenomatosis, and 3 to 5 years in the case of maedi.

Note: All older sheep which are 'thin for teeth', i.e. they have body scores below that of their contemporaries on adequate nutritional inputs, and without evidence of tooth disease, can be presumed to have a high probability of chronic respiratory disease, and culling should be considered.

Acute dyspnoea (upper respiratory tract)

- Check for laryngeal chondritis (oedema and obstruction) – particularly common in Texels but also seen in other short necked breeds.

Chronic dyspnoea (upper respiratory 'snoring')

This may result from O. ovis infection, chronic infection of nasal passages, tumours, but antemortem diagnosis is likely to prove difficult.

Radiography may be considered in the case of a valuable animal.

Postmortem diagnosis of respiratory disease

The vast majority of sheep suffering overwhelming respiratory disorders also suffer 'sudden death' or more accurately 'found dead'. It follows that accurate diagnosis depends on competence in the technique of carrying out a postmortem examination, and in the selection of the correct samples, together with their preservation and transit (see appendices).

It must be borne in mind that with the possible exception of SPA, MV, and perhaps the septicaemic form of pasteurellosis, postmortem lesions are not pathognomonic (see Figure 21.1). Accurate diagnosis depends on observation plus bacteriological and histological examinations.

Gross pathology

Note: It has been stated that by the time a sheep has died it is too late for a postmortem examination! Although this is an

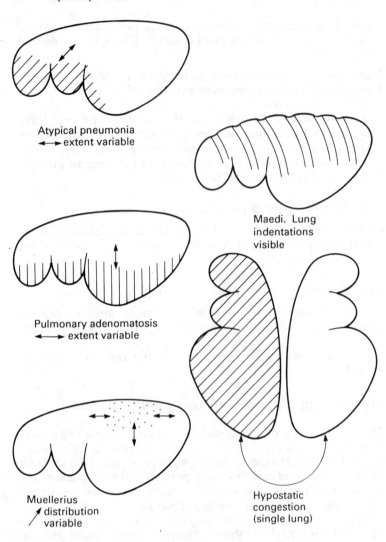

Figure 21.1 Distribution of lesions in respiratory disease

overstatement, the effect of the fleece in delaying heat loss after death, together with possible extremes of pyrexia in the final stages of infective conditions often give accelerated autolysis with severe limitations on the value of single necropsies.

Neonate (see also chapter 8)

- Check for initial expansion of lungs.
  Apparent consolidation, sinks in water, indicates stillbirth.
  Apparent consolidation but neutral gravity, indicates neonatal acute respiratory distress syndrome.
  Apparent lobular consolidation indicates incomplete expansion.
  Floats in water indicates full expansion.
- Check for pleural haemorrhage; indicates parturient trauma.
- Check for miliary abscess formation; indicates neonatal septicaemia.
- Check for anterior lobe consolidation and fluid in bronchioles; indicates inhalation pneumonia.
- Check for congestion; indicates possible acute pasteurellosis/viral infection. (If only one lung affected, may be hypostatic congestion.)

Note: At this age, pasteurellosis is usually septicaemic. Check for generalized septicaemia lesions – petechiation of epicardium, spleen, liver, kidneys and hyperaemia of abdominal and thoracic lymph nodes.

Growing lambs

The gross appearance of any lung tissue which has been subject to delay between death and examination, will frequently show a degree of reddening due to early autolysis, which is easily confused with the changes shown in early pasteurellosis. In the case of the latter, there is more likely to be some fluid in the airways, and possibly evidence of generalized infection in other parts of the carcase.

Uniform congestion with darkened colour

- Check for peracute pasteurellosis (isolation and quantification of organisms from piece of lung tissue, plus histology).
- Check for delay between death and examination – autolysis.

Lobular consolidation – apical and cardiac lobes

- Check for inhalation pneumonia (history).
- Check for viral pneumonia.
- Check for atypical pneumonia (histology).
- Check for other chronic infection, abscessation.

Lobular consolidation – random

- Check for atypical pneumonia – grey to red *raised* areas.
- Check for chronic pasteurellosis – edges discrete, possible necrosis, surface *sunken*.
- Check for after effects of neonatal septicaemia – abscesses and chronic change at the interface with normal tissue.
- Check for parasitic pneumonia – emphysema and oedema, presence of worms in bronchi.

Subpleural nodules in caudal lobes

- Check for *M. capillaris* (incidental finding only).

Single lung congestion

- Check for hypostatic congestion, recumbency before death (may be other signs such as excoriation of limb or eye region).

Petechiation

- Check upper respiratory tract for similar lesions, suggests peracute pasteurellosis.
- Check for Biotype T septicaemias – usually appears as death of a number of animals in autumn.

Pleurisy
This lesion is likely to accompany any infectious and febrile pneumonic condition, and the extent and degree of pleurisy will be an indication of the duration of the infection.

- Pleural cavity full of straw coloured fluid with fibrin clots suggests peracute pasteurellosis.
- Thick green gelatinous exudate suggests subacute pasteurellosis.
- Total or near total occlusion of pleural cavity with widespread adhesions suggests chronic pasteurellosis.
- Fibrinous tags associated with clearly demarcated areas of consolidation suggests atypical pneumonia.

Adults

Many of the comments in the previous section will apply to this age group, but the important slow viral conditions will also feature prominently. Where lesions of acute pasteurellosis are found, a careful examination should be made for lesions of pulmonary adenomatosis since these can easily be missed.

Lungs larger than normal

- Check for areas of pulmonary adenomatosis tumour (vary in size from 0.5 cm to involvement of up to half diaphragmatic lobe) – solid, grey or purple in colour, clearly demarcated from normal lung unless masked by generalized pneumonia. Excess fluid in airways.

Lungs do not collapse, rib impressions visible

- Check for maedi visna (histology, serology).

Petechiae in upper respiratory tract

- Check for septicaemic form of pasteurellosis.

Inflammation and swelling of pharyngeal and laryngeal area

- Check for breed – laryngeal chondritis in Texels.
- Check for tracks from drenching injury.

Bronchial froth and fluid
This will accompany many conditions, even postmortem change. If excessive:

- Check for parasitic bronchitis.
- Check for inhalation pneumonia.
- Check for pulmonary adenomatosis.

As previously stated, with respiratory disorders confirmation of any causal organism or parasites will depend on laboratory tests such as microbiology, histology and parasitology.

It must be noted that *P. haemolytica* is a normal inhabitant of the upper respiratory tract, and that to establish this as a cause of pneumonia lesions it is necessary to isolate in large numbers from the lesion itself.

PI3 may also be isolated from the upper respiratory tract, but this does not necessarily indicate a direct involvement in any disease process.

22 Sudden death

Accident
Lightning strike
Trauma
Predation
Neonatal deaths
Young lambs
Growing and store lambs
Adults
Abdominal catastrophe
Metabolic disease
Acute infections
Parasitism
Toxins

Because of the nature of stock supervision in the sheep industry – at best twice daily in the lowland unit and infrequently in the high hill unit, what appears to be sudden death is usually simply death since the last inspection. It should, therefore, be more accurately described as 'found dead'. Apart from true sudden death caused by accidents, trauma or lightning strike, and some overwhelming bacterial infections, few deaths will be asymptomatic as presented by the owner, who may not wish to admit that he has not examined the stock as often or as thoroughly as he should.

Postmortem examination (the technique of which is described in Appendix 1) will obviously play a central role in any 'found dead' investigation. However, the rapid onset of autolysis, hastened by the presence of the fleece which delays cooling of the carcase, poses limitations on the value of this examination unless the time lapse is reasonably short. It has been said that the only valuable PME in the sheep is one carried out before death!

It is therefore essential to obtain a full history, and if there is any suggestion of a flock problem, to examine thoroughly contact animals for any less advanced cases.

A record of findings should be kept, but if there is any possibility of insurance claims or legal action, it is essential that careful and comprehensive details are kept.

The age and sex of the animal will exclude some conditions. Other important aspects in the history taking include:

• grazing history
• feeding, roughage and concentrates, especially recent changes
• vaccination history, any recent vaccination
• recent drenching, with what? how much?
• other recent stress – dipping, shearing, weaning
• recent close confinement.

Although suggestions are made of the most likely causes of 'sudden death' or 'found dead' in various age categories, this does not imply that other causes do not exist nor that a thorough PME need not be carried out!

Sudden death at any age

Obviously accidents, lightning strike and trauma are no respecters of age.

Accidents

Accidents should be capable of diagnosis even if not witnessed, but it is necessary to beware of the 'contrived' accident where no external or internal evidence can be found, particularly where an insurance claim is involved.

Lightning strike

Lightning strike is also a popular candidate for insurance claims, often with considerable client pressure exerted. If lightning is suspected (by the clinician not just by the owner), then the circumstances of death must be investigated.

- Check weather at time of incident – with local meteorological office if necessary.
- Check the site for adjacent trees/buildings/ metal fences.
- Check for scorching of grass.
- Check for evidence of external singeing or burns.
- Check for subcutaneous haemorrhages, sometimes in a branching pattern.
- Other PM signs are not diagnostic, therefore a final diagnosis must rest on a combination of circumstances and signs.

Trauma

Trauma, particularly by predators such as dogs is another common occurrence, again possibly involving insurance or legal aspects.

- Check carefully that injury was inflicted before death – there should be signs of bruising or haemorrhage into tissues adjacent to injury.
- Check for puncture wounds and other tooth marks, again with signs of bruising.
- Predation is common once an animal has died, if not removed immediately, and it is not unknown for an unscrupulous owner to attempt to simulate predation on an already dead animal.

Common causes of 'sudden death' or 'found dead'

Neonatal lambs

For full details see chapter 8. Most lamb deaths in the first few days after birth will be 'found dead' rather than true sudden deaths. Because of their susceptibility to hypothermia, however, the period during which symptoms of illness may be seen is likely to be short.

Common causes are: trauma, overlying/suffocation, exposure, starvation, lamb dysentery, neonatal septicaemia.

Young lambs (milk dependent)

The most common cause of death in this age group is starvation, which, by definition, is not sudden death although the owner may think so!

- Check ewe milk supply.
- Check body fat reserves in lamb.
- Check abomasum for presence of milk.
- Check for disease predisposing to starvation, e.g. orf, neonatal polyarthritis, neonatal septicaemia.
- Check for nephrosis – there should be some warning signs, but where very young lambs are affected death can occur quickly.

Other causes of death

Individual lambs dead

There are a small number of abdominal conditions in this age group which can cause rapid death.

- Check for 'red gut', i.e. torsion of the mesentery involving the intestines except the first part of the duodenum. If seen alive, lambs are bloated and deteriorate over a very short time (30 min). PME shows very distended dark red intestines, and the site of the twist can be identified. This may be seen in lambs at grass, but is probably more common in artificially fed or creep fed lambs. It is thought to be due to rapid passage of rich gas-producing food into the intestine producing instability of the intestines, which then twist irreversibly, occluding the anterior mesenteric artery.
- Check for gastric torsion – this occasionally occurs in lambs before rumen development has begun.
- Bloat of either the abomasum, or when developed, the rumen may occur, usually in artificially fed lambs. Unless the lamb is seen alive with bloat, it is difficult to be sure whether bloating occurred before or after death.

Many lambs dead

Probably the most common cause of well-nourished lambs being 'found dead' is peracute pasteurellosis (biotype A). This often occurs at 3–4 weeks of age as maternal antibody wanes.

- Check for signs of septicaemia – petechiae of heart, liver, spleen and kidneys, swelling and hyperaemia of cervical and thoracic lymph nodes. There is often no pneumonia or pleurisy in this young age group. Diagnosis can be confirmed by submitting a selection of tissues for bacteriological examination.
- Check also for acute abomasitis. *P. haemolytica* has been isolated from the mucosa but not from other organs in these cases.

The beginning of outbreaks of severe coccidiosis and/or nematodiriasis may be signalled by lambs 'found dead', but careful examination of the remainder of the group should reveal others showing clinical signs of infection (see chapter 10).

- Check for lesions of coccidiosis in lower small intestine, caecum and colon – raised white spots, mucosa thickened and inflamed. Smears of intestinal scrapings show developing stages of coccidia.
- Check for immature *Nematodirus* in small intestine – slender worms about 2 cm long which when coiled together can look like cottonwool.

Growing and store lambs

In this group, sporadic deaths can occur from a variety of causes, but the most important conditions are those which cause a series of deaths if not diagnosed initially and preventive measures taken.

Individual lambs dead

- Check for abdominal catastrophe – red gut or other acute obstruction.
- In males, check for unobserved urolithiasis and ruptured bladder.
- Check for nephrosis.
- If recently drenched, check for dosing gun injury.
- If recently dipped, check for inhalation pneumonia.
- Check heart muscle for white streaks (nutritional myopathy).

Many lambs dead

Changes in feeding often trigger flock outbreaks of disease in this age group. This is particularly true of pulpy kidney which usually follows change to lush pasture, or sudden grass growth after rain. There is also a suggestion that pasteurellosis follows feed changes.

- Check for systemic pasteurellosis (biotype T). Characteristic necrotic lesions of the tongue, pharynx, oesophagus and sometimes the abomasum and intestine are usually present, together with subcutaneous and subpleural haemorrhages, enlargement of tonsils and retropharyngeal lymph nodes, and necrotic foci in liver and spleen. Take samples of lesions and swabs of ulcerations for bacteriological examination. Diagnosis is confirmed by isolation of large numbers of *P. haemolytica* and serotyping.
- Check for pulpy kidney (enterotoxaemia caused by *Clostridium perfringens* type D, Table 22.1) – in fresh carcase, kidneys are pale and swollen, but autolysis is rapid giving the disease its name. Other findings are excess pericardial fluid, and haemorrhages in the heart. Smears can be made of small intestine and kidney for FAT. Check also urine sample for presence of glucose (there is usually sufficient to moisten a test stick even if the bladder appears empty).

Table 22.1 Clostridial diseases causing rapid death

Disease	Organism	Age group affected	Predisposing factors
Lamb dysentery	Cl. perfringens type B	Neonatal lambs <2 weeks	Unvaccinated ewes
Pulpy kidney	Cl. perfringens type D	Growing lambs	Waning maternal immunity Fast growing lambs Lush grass
Braxy	Cl. septicum (chauvoei type A)	Store lambs	Unvaccinated Frozen foods
Black disease	Cl. oedematiens type B	Store lambs Adults	Unvaccinated Migrating liver fluke
Struck	Cl. perfringens type C	Adults	Unvaccinated Lush grass
Blackleg	Cl. chauvoei type B	Growing lambs and adults	Unvaccinated, Wounds, injuries

- Check vaccination history. Maternal antibody wanes after 12–16 weeks. Many lambs are unprotected after this age, or receive a single vaccination which is inadequate to ensure full protection.
- In frosty weather, check for braxy (*Cl. septicum*) (Table 22.1). PME shows acute inflammation of the abomasum, excess fluid in the abdomen, and rapid autolysis. Confirm diagnosis by FAT on smear from abomasal lesion.
- If fed concentrates, or access to concentrates or grain, check for acidosis – examine rumen contents for undigested foodstuffs, and check pH (normal is 5.5, less than 4.5 indicates cereal overeating).
- Check for acute liver fluke especially in wet season if grazing poorly drained land. Acute disease occurs about 6 weeks after ingestion of large numbers of metacercariae. PME shows enlarged liver with haemorrhagic tracts, often covered with fibrinous exudate, blood-stained fluid in abdomen. In unvaccinated flocks, there may also be cases of black disease (Table 22.1) (*Cl. oedematiens* type B) – rapid putrefaction, oedema of abdominal wall, dark engorged liver with areas of necrosis.
  Check remainder of group for clinical cases – anaemia, enlarged painful abdomens.
- Check for other acute parasitic infection – *Nematodirus*, *Haemonchus*, *Ostertagia*. In each of these cases, the observant shepherd should note warning signs before deaths occur.

Adults

Although a large proportion of ewe deaths occur in the periparturient period (see chapter 6), there is still a wide variety of conditions which may kill ewes or rams at any time of year. It is important again to emphasize the difference between 'sudden death' and 'found dead', and an assessment of the body condition of the animal will usually give a good guide to the presence of disease of some duration. Other vital pieces of evidence are:

- position of carcase when found,
- access to poisonous plants, mouth contents,
- vaccination history,
- recent feeding or management changes,
- recent handling, e.g. shearing, dipping, drenching.

Note: Although anthrax rarely appears to be identified as a cause of sudden death in sheep, the possibility should not be totally ignored, especially if a very enlarged spleen is found during PME.

Individual deaths

Probably the most common cause is 'cast on back', i.e. the sheep is in such a position that it cannot sit or stand up. This most often affects fat sheep in heavy fleece, and bloat is usually the actual cause of death. There is always a pile of faeces behind the animal, indicating the length of time for which it was lying in that position. It is essential to see the carcase *in situ*, in order to make a valid judgement as to whether this was likely to be the cause of death.

If recently handled for dipping, shearing, drenching, vaccination, etc.

- Check for sudden catastrophe, e.g. ruptured major blood vessel, heart lesion.
- Check for precipitation of metabolic disease (hypocalcaemia, hypomagnesaemia – see below).

If lactating ewe

- Check for acute (gangrenous) mastitis.
- Check for hypomagnesaemia – see below.

If one of group of rams

- Check for broken neck caused by fighting. This is particularly common at the beginning of the breeding season, or when new rams are introduced. It may also occur in an established group after shearing or dipping.
- Check for clostridial infection of wounds from fighting, i.e. head wounds.

Many deaths

Where deaths are occurring in sufficient numbers to constitute a flock problem, the causes fall most commonly into four categories:

- Bacterial (*Clostridia, Pasteurella*)
- Metabolic (hypocalcaemia, hypomagnesaemia)
- Parasitic (acute fluke, *Haemonchus*)
- Toxic (copper, plants).

Significant numbers of ewe deaths have also been reported after prelambing vaccination.

If deaths follow vaccination

- Check vaccination technique, sterility of equipment, use of new needles.
- Check for use of previously opened vaccine packs.
- Check for vaccinating wet or dirty animals.
- Check for concurrent metabolic disease, e.g. hypocalcaemia, pregnancy toxaemia – these may have been precipitated by temporary removal from food source, or handling.
- Check for concurrent administration of anthelmintic, flukicide. It may be advisable not to administer more than one drug at a time.
- Check for true hypersensitivity reaction – pulmonary oedema and pleural effusion may suggest this. Consult manufacturer.

If no obvious lesions found at PME

- Check for metabolic disease – hypocalcaemia is most commonly seen in late pregnancy, hypomagnesaemia in early lactation especially ewes on lush pasture rearing twins. Aqueous humour is useful for sampling and should be stable for up to 48 h. Cerebrospinal fluid may also be used and is stable for up to 12 h after death.

Note: Hypocalcaemia can occur occasionally at times other than late pregnancy, and in non-pregnant animals, and is precipitated by severe stress, e.g. long transport, driving long distances.

If lung lesions found

- Check for acute pasteurellosis (see chapter 21). Care must be taken to distinguish between hypostatic congestion and pneumonia, but in acute pasteurellosis areas of necrosis are often found in consolidated areas of lung, and pleurisy and pericarditis are usually present. Confirmation requires isolation of large numbers of organisms from lung tissue, and histological examination.
- Check for masking of lesions of pulmonary adenomatosis especially if animal is in poor condition.

If liver lesions are found

- Check for acute liver fluke (see above).

- Check for black disease in conjunction with acute fluke (see above).
- If jaundice is present, check for copper poisoning (see chapter 18).

If carcase is pale and oedematous

- Check abomasum for *Haemonchus contortus*. Worms are easily visible (2–3 cm), plus haemorrhagic gastritis.

If autolysis is very rapid

- Check for clostridial disease (vaccination history?).

Struck (*Cl. perfringens* type C) shows excess abdominal fluid, hyperaemia and ulceration of small intestine. Confirm by smear for FAT or toxin neutralization test with intestinal contents.

Blackleg (*Cl. chauvoei*) features acute necrotizing myositis. Often the site of the main lesion can be identified by crepitus from gas in the tissues which are dark red and haemorrhagic with a characteristic rancid smell. Diagnosis is confirmed by FAT on smears or frozen sections of affected tissue.

If plant poisoning is suspected

- Check mouth contents – yew causes true 'sudden death' by the action of the alkaloid taxine, which acts directly on the heart.
- Check rumen contents – remains of plants such as rhododendron or acorns may be visible. Neither of these kill instantaneously so symptoms of illness should be seen in others exposed to same environment.

Note: Rhododendron poisoning is the most likely cause of 'vomiting' in sheep. (Excess intake of linseed meal, and acidosis have also been reported as causes of vomiting.)

Other toxins which may cause death

- Brassicas may cause haemolytic anaemia.
- High nitrate content in kale may cause nitrite poisoning (nitrate is converted to nitrite in the rumen). The distinguishing feature is methaemoglobinaemia.
- Acute lead poisoning – death is usually preceded by fits. PME shows grey musculature, liver degeneration, and gastroenteritis. Submit liver and kidney for analysis.
- Phenols present in some dips, disinfectants, creosote, etc. are

toxic, and can often be detected in a carcase by smell. Signs of an irritant poison are present if ingestion has occurred, or severe pneumonia if incorrect dipping has taken place. Samples for analysis should include stomach contents, lung, liver, kidney, urine and blood. If immediate transport to a laboratory cannot be arranged, samples can be frozen.

Appendix 1
Postmortem
examination

It is either an indictment of the sheep industry, or a reflection of the 'death wish' of sheep, that a considerable amount of disease diagnosis in this species depends on material obtained at PME for a final verdict. However, this is often an undervalued technique in practice, carried out in a cursory 'slash and glance' manner, stopping when one gross lesion is found. It *should* be carried out in a careful, scientific and logical manner, so that all organs are examined in order to gain maximum information, and to select samples which give the greatest opportunity to obtain a correct diagnosis. It must be stressed that any PME should be performed as soon after death as possible, if autolytic change is not to complicate or mask any pathological change.

Stages in a postmortem examination

(1) External examination (Figure A1.1)
Identity
Age
Sex
Weight
Time since death
Body condition
Fleece state
Mouth, nose, eyes, mucous membrane
Udder, vulva/scrotum, prepuce
Anus

Note: Discoloration of the ventral abdomen is not an indication of infection, simply of autolysis, which may be evident within 24 h of death, or earlier in hot weather.

(2) Place the animal on its back, or on its side (this is easier with a thin animal). Cut through and reflect the skin from mandible to pubis. Cut into axilla and groin on both sides if on back, or on upper side if on side, to free the close attachments of the legs (Figure A1.2).
(3) Examine subcutis, superficial lymph nodes, udder or penis and testicles.
(4) Cut through abdominal wall, taking care to avoid puncturing the rumen, and expose abdominal organs. Examine *in situ*. Note amount of fat in mesentery.
(5) Cut through ribs along each side with saw or shears to expose thoracic organs. Examine *in situ* (Figure A1.3).
(6) Remove alimentary tract by cutting through rectum and

213

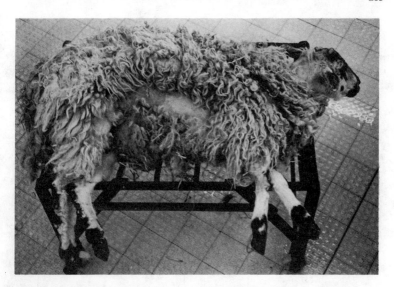

Figure A1.1 External examination

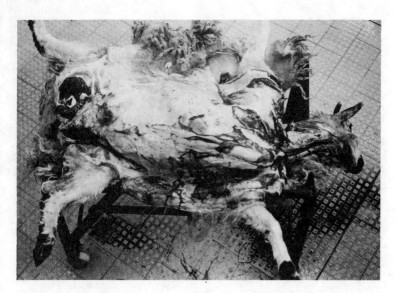

Figure A1.2 Subcutaneous tissues exposed, legs reflected

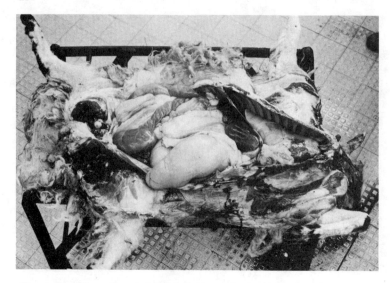

Figure A1.3 Thoracic and abdominal viscera *in situ* (omentum removed)

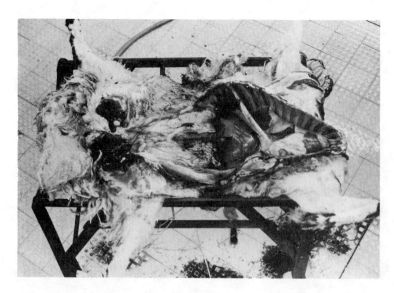

Figure A1.4 Gastrointestinal tract removed, leaving liver, kidneys and uterus

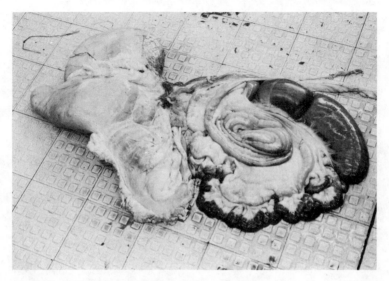

Figure A1.5 Gastrointestinal tract

separating from roof of abdominal cavity forward until oesophagus can be cut through as it passes through diaphragm (Figure A1.4). Place organs to one side (Figure A1.5).

(7) Remove liver and spleen and place to one side.

(8) Cut inside mandibles to free tongue, reflect with oesophagus and trachea, and remove with lungs and heart. Put to one side (Figure A1.6).

(9) Examine pleural cavity.

(10) Cut through cheeks and disarticulate jaw, examine incisor and molar teeth.

(11) Examine and remove uterus if present.

(12) Examine and remove kidneys. Note amount of perirenal fat. Examine bladder, collect urine if necessary.

(13) Examine and open several joints.

(14) Return to thoracic organs. Open oesophagus, trachea and bronchi. Examine mediastinal lymph nodes. Palpate and cut into lung substance. Open pericardium. Open both sides of heart and great vessels.

(15) Return to abdominal organs. Separate rumen, reticulum and omasum from abomasum. Open, examine contents and save if necessary. Wash and examine mucosa.

216

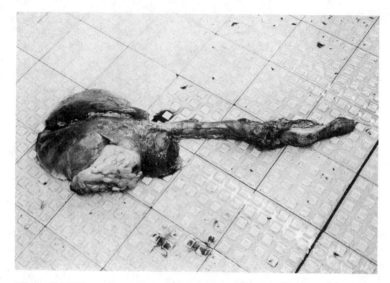

Figure A1.6 Thoracic organs, with trachea, oesophagus and tongue

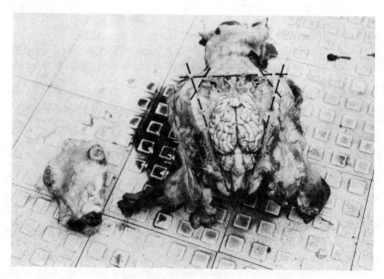

Figure A1.7 Head with brain exposed. Sawmarks superimposed

(16) Separate abomasum from duodenum. Open, examine contents, save if necessary. Wash mucosa and examine.

(17) Examine small intestine, caecum and colon. Open, save contents if necessary, examine mucosa.

(18) Examine mesenteric lymph nodes.

(19) Examine and incise liver, spleen and kidneys.

(20) Remove head by disarticulating atlanto-occipital joint. Reflect skin. Make cuts with saw as indicated in Figure A1.7. Lever off top of skull. Reflect dura, and free tentorium cerebelli. Invert, and carefully remove whole brain. Examine surface but do not cut into substance until fixed.

Agonal and postmortem change

Agonal changes take place immediately before death, and are due to circulatory failure. The most common change of which to beware in this category is hypostatic congestion of the lower lung, which may be confused with pneumonia. If there is any doubt, a sample of lung tissue should be taken for bacteriology and histology (including quantification of *Pasteurella* – see chapter 21).

If barbiturates are used for euthanasia, parts of the small intestine are often found to be dilated and congested.

The most rapid postmortem change in sheep is bloat, which develops rapidly, making a diagnosis of death from bloat extremely difficult.

Decomposition is rapid in warm weather, or if the animal has a heavy fleece. In cold weather it will be much slower, making PME useful for a longer period after death. If clostridial infection is involved, decomposition will be rapid anyway.

Checklist of organs

External examination, wool, skin.
Subcutaneous tissue.
Alimentary tract – teeth, tongue, oesophagus, rumen, reticulum, omasum, abomasum, small intestine, caecum, large intestine, anus.
Respiratory system – larynx, trachea, bronchi, lungs, pleura.
Cardiovascular system – pericardium, heart.
Urinary system – kidneys, bladder, urethra.

Genital system – uterus, ovaries, fetuses and placenta if present, vagina, vulva, udder/scrotum, testicles, penis, prepuce.
Musculoskeletal system – muscles, joints, feet.
Lymphoid system – spleen, lymph nodes, bone marrow.
Nervous system – meninges, brain, spinal cord, eyes.

Appendix 2
Sample taking/sample sending

Submission of incorrect samples is a waste of time and money for the client and the clinician, and may result in the loss of potentially valuable material from the point of view of diagnosis. Many laboratories now supply kits of sample containers, transport media, etc., and will be only too pleased to give advice on sample submission if asked. If any unusual samples or requests are to be submitted prior consultation is essential.

Packing and posting samples

Written details with practice name, identity of the animal, owner, history, and specific requests for tests required should be enclosed in a polythene bag for protection. Post Office regulations state that pathological specimens should be enclosed in a sealed receptacle which itself should be securely enclosed in a strong outer container so that it cannot move about. If necessary, the receptacle should be enclosed in a polythene bag with a sufficient quantity of absorbent material to prevent possible leakage. The packet should be marked *Fragile with care* and *Pathological specimen*, and should be sent by first class post, not parcel post. Any packet not packed and marked as above, or found in parcel post will be destroyed. Anyone not complying with these regulations is liable to prosecution.

Samples for haematology

EDTA is the anticoagulant of choice. Heparin and OxF are not suitable for a full haematological examination. Care should be taken to use the correct size of container for the volume of blood to be collected, i.e. don't put a small volume of blood in a large vacutainer, as the excess of anticoagulant can distort the results.

Samples for enzymology

Serum or plasma (with heparin as anticoagulant) are suitable for most tests, except where red cell enzymes (GSH-Px, SOD, TK) are to be measured, when a heparinized sample is essential. If a clotted blood sample is obtained, it is preferable to separate the serum before submission, as haemolysis may interfere with the tests. Samples should be submitted as quickly as possible (certainly in less than 36h), since some enzymes have a short life. SDH must be assayed within 4h of collection.

Enzymes which may be helpful in ovine clinical diagnosis

Creatine kinase (CK)
This is raised in skeletal muscle damage, e.g. in nutritional myopathy (muscular dystrophy, white muscle disease). However, this enzyme has a short half-life within the body, therefore sampling should be done early in the course of a disease.

Aspartate aminotransferase (AST)
Raised in muscle damage, and acute liver damage, but needs other tests to support.

Glutamate dehydrogenase (GLDH)
Raised in hepatitis. In conjunction with raised AST indicates acute liver damage.

Gamma glutamyl transferase (GGT)
Raised in chronic hepatitis, particularly with bile duct damage, e.g. chronic liver fluke. May also be raised in cases of pregnancy toxaemia.

Sorbitol dehydrogenase (SDH)
Raised in acute hepatitis and is liver specific. *Must* be assayed within 4h of sampling.

Requiring heparinized blood

Glutathione peroxidase (GSH-Px)
Is used as an indicator of selenium (vitamin E) status.

Superoxide dismutase (SOD)
Is an indicator of prolonged copper deficiency.

Transketolase (TK)
Is a specific indicator for CCN.

Samples for biochemistry

These are most likely to be helpful on a flock rather than on an individual basis. A minimum of six samples from representative animals should be collected. In the case of individual animals suffering from a suspected metabolic disease, it may be wise to collect pre-treatment blood samples which will then be available in the event of failure to respond to treatment.

Tests requiring serum or plasma (heparinized)

Calcium, magnesium, beta-hydroxybutyrate, urea, creatinine, total protein, albumin, globulin, copper, vitamin B_{12}.

Tests requiring anticoagulant (potassium oxalate/sodium fluoride)

Inorganic phosphorus, glucose.

Aqueous humour or CSF may be useful in dead animals, especially for calcium and magnesium estimation.

Samples for bacteriology

Fresh samples should be taken and submitted as quickly as possible. Pieces of tissue, e.g. liver, spleen, lung, lymph node, etc. should be placed in sterile containers. If swabs are to be used these should be of cottonwool, with, if possible, transport medium (without antibiotics). Unprotected swabs dry out and are useless – these should be placed in a protective container. *Mycoplasma*, *Campylobacter*, *Leptospira* and *Chlamydia* (unless in placenta) have particular requirements – contact laboratory for advice before sending.

If anaerobes are suspected, air should be excluded from samples by wrapping with clingfilm. If *Clostridia* are suspected, dried smears of lesions may be useful for FAT.

Samples for virology

Take advice from laboratory except for
Orf – dried scab
Border disease – blood clot (keep cool and rapid submission), nasal swab in virus transport medium, serum from affected and contact animals.
Rotavirus – faeces sample (rectal swab is not adequate).

Samples for serology

Single samples are useless, except with EAE where a high post-abortion titre is significant. In other cases paired sera are required, but the first sample must be taken early in the disease process, otherwise seroconversion may have already taken place.

Samples for abortion enquiry

A representative number of samples from an affected flock should be submitted, i.e. at least 10% of abortions.

Whole placenta or piece of placenta with cotyledons from an area showing pathological change, if present.

Fetus(es) or vacutainer of stomach contents plus vacutainer of pleural fluid plus piece of fetal liver.

Vaginal swab if placenta not available.

Serum sample may be helpful in some cases. Aborting ewes should be marked so that a blood sample can be obtained later if required.

Samples for histology

Take small pieces of fresh tissue less than 1 cm thick (except in the case of brain which should be left whole) and place in a wide-mouthed container (if a narrow container is used it may be impossible to remove the fixed sample without breaking it – the container or the sample!). Use about 20 parts fixative to 1 part of tissue to ensure rapid penetration.

A suitable fixative is 10% neutral buffered formalin:

100 ml formaldehyde 40% (formalin)
900 ml distilled water
6.5 g disodium hydrogen phosphate (anhydrous)
  4 g sodium dihydrogen phosphate monohydrate
or formol saline:
100 ml formaldehyde 40% (formalin)
  9 g sodium chloride
900 ml tap water.

Samples for toxicology

Consult laboratory if any unusual toxin is suspected. Take particular care if the case is of a nature where litigation may be involved. In this case, duplicate samples should be taken and placed in containers which are sealed in the presence of a witness, if possible.

Helpful samples may include

Blood (oxalated) and faeces from live animals.

Stomach contents, liver, kidney, brain, fat, muscle from PME.

Food material if suspected (1 kg if available).

Any suspected poison source.

For copper poisoning take liver and kidney (100 g).

For fluorine take urine and bone (tail or rib).

For lead take liver and kidney (100 g).

For molybdenum take liver (100 g).

For organophosphorus/chlorine compounds take brain, fat, stomach contents, liver and kidney.

For monensin, take food sample plus contents label.

Samples for parasitology

For worm egg counts, fluke egg counts and coccidial oocyst counts, 10 g of faeces in a plastic container is required for each test. Counts may be carried out on smaller amounts, but these may be less accurate. However, it is realized that there are practical difficulties in obtaining large amounts from small scouring lambs!

For worm counts, it may be easiest to deliver the whole of the alimentary tract (suitably ligated at each end). It is possible to empty out separately the contents of the abomasum and small intestine, but these require washing through to make sure that all worms have been harvested. A small amount of formol saline should be added if the samples are not to be delivered to the laboratory on the day of collection.

For cryptosporidia, 5 g of faeces in a plastic container is required.

For abomasal parasitism, pepsinogen can be measured with 7 ml clotted blood.

For skin conditions, macroscopically visible parasites should be submitted in a clean dry bottle.

For ringworm and *Dermatophilus* infections, scabs, skin scrapings, and fibres from the edge of an active lesion should be submitted in a clean dry bottle.

Appendix 3
Standard reference values

Note: The following values are for guidance only. 'Normal' values may vary slightly according to the test method used (especially in the case of enzymes). The guidance of the particular laboratory performing the test should always be followed.

Haematology

RBC 5–12 × 10^{12}/l
Hb 8–15 g/dl
PCV 0.24–0.40
MCV 25–40 fl
MCHC 31–36 g/dl
Reticulocytes 0%
WBC Total 4–12 × 10^9/l
Lymphocytes 2–9 × 10^9/l (40–75%)
Neutrophils 0.5–6 × 10^9/l (10–50%)
Monocytes 0–0.7 × 10^9/l (0–6%)
Eosinophils 0–1 × 10^9/l (0–10%)
Basophils 0–0.5 × 10^9/l (0–3%)

Enzymology

CK <50 i.u./l
AST <60 i.u./l
GLDH <2 i.u./l
GGT <30 i.u./l
SDH <5 i.u./l
GSH-Px >40 i.u./ml RBCs (Se equivalent >1.3 μmol/l) is adequate
        <13 i.u./ml RBCs (Se equivalent <0.6 μmol/l) is deficient
SOD >0.4 i.u./mg Hb in lambs, >0.3 i.u./mg Hb in ewes
TK >90 i.u./ml RBCs indicates CCN. <12 indicates not CCN.

Biochemistry

Ca 2–3 mmol/l
Inorganic P 1–2.5 mmol/l
Mg 0.7–1.5 mmol/l
Cu 10–20 μmol/l
Vitamin B_{12} (Co) >0.15 pmol/ml
Se >1.3 μmol/l is adequate, <0.6 μmol/l is deficient

Urea 3–8 mmol/l
Creatine <150 µmol/l
Glucose 2–3 mmol/l
BHB <1 µmol/l
Bilirubin <10 µmol/l
Total protein 60–80 g/l
Albumin 25–35 g/l
IgG 25–40 g/l
Pepsinogen <1 i.u./l

Sources

Diseases of Sheep. Ed. W.B. Martin, Blackwell, Oxford
Veterinary Laboratory Data. B. Rushton. BVA publications
Schalms Veterinary Haematology, 4th Edn. N.C. Jain. Lea and Febiger, New York
Veterinary Laboratory Medicine. M.G. Kerr. Blackwell, Oxford
In Practice. D. Jones. Vol. 10, 1988, 241–244.

Appendix 4
Abbreviations

AST	aspartate aminotransferase	IHA	indirect haemagglutination
BD	border disease	LAT	latex agglutination test
BHB	beta hydroxybutyrate		
Ca	Calcium	Mg	magnesium
CCN	cerebrocortical necrosis	MJ	megajoules
		MV	maedi visna
CFT	complement fixation test	OxF	oxalate fluoride
		P	phosphorus
CK	creatine kinase	PCV	packed cell volume
Co	cobalt	PGE	parasitic gastroenteritis
CSF	cerebrospinal fluid		
DM	dry matter	PI3	parainfluenzae 3 virus
DVO	Divisional Veterinary Officer		
		PME	postmortem examination
EAE	enzootic abortion of ewes	PMSG	pregnant mares' serum gonadotrophin
EDTA	ethylene diamine tetra-acetic acid	POM	prescription only medicine
ELISA	enzyme-linked immunosorbent assay		
		RBC	red blood cells
EM	electron microscopy	SAT	serum agglutination test
ETEC	enterotoxigenic *E. coli*		
FAT	fluorescent antibody test	SDH	sorbitol dehydrogenase
		SOD	superoxide dismutase
GGT	gamma glutamyl transferase	SPA	sheep pulmonary adenomatosis
GLDH	glutamate dehydrogenase	SORP	suboptimal reproductive performance
GSH-Px	glutathione peroxidase		
		TK	transketolase
HAT	haemagglutination test	UDP	undegradable protein
		WBC	white blood cells
Hb	haemoglobin	ZN	Ziehl Neelson
IFAT	indirect fluorescent antibody test		

Further reading

Books

Arthur, G.H., Noakes, D.E. and Pearson, H. *Veterinary Reproduction and Obstetrics*, 7th Edition (1989) Bailliere Tindall, London

Blood, D.C. and Brightling, D.P. *Veterinary Information Management* (1989) Bailliere Tindall, London

Blood, D.C. and Radostits, O.M. *Veterinary Medicine*, 7th Edition (1989) Bailliere Tindall, London

Clarkson, M.J. and Faull, W.B. *A Handbook for the Sheep Clinician*, 4th Edition (1989) Liverpool University Press, Liverpool

Fraser, A. and Stamp, J.T. *Sheep Husbandry and Diseases*, 6th Edition (1987) Collins, London

Marai, I., Fayez, M. and Owen, J.B. (Eds) *New Techniques in Sheep Production* (1987) Butterworths, London

Martin, W.B. (Ed.) *Diseases of Sheep*, 2nd Edition (1990) Blackwell Scientific Publications, Oxford

Oliver, J.E., Hoerlein, B.F. and Mayhew, I.G. *Veterinary Neurology* (1987) W.B. Saunders, New York

Publications

Proceedings of the Sheep Veterinary Society (annually)
In Practice (Supplement to the *Veterinary Record*) (bimonthly)

Tape/slide programmes

Boundy, T. *Care and Examination of Rams*. VET 41 Unit for Continuing Veterinary Education, Royal Veterinary College

Linklater, K.A. *Infectious Abortion in Sheep*. VET 37 Unit for Continuing Veterinary Education, Royal Veterinary College

Index

Note: page numbers in *italics* refer to figures and tables

236   Index